KETO
MEAL PREP

*Easy Recipes to Burn Body Fat and
Get Back in Good Shape*

MAX LOREN

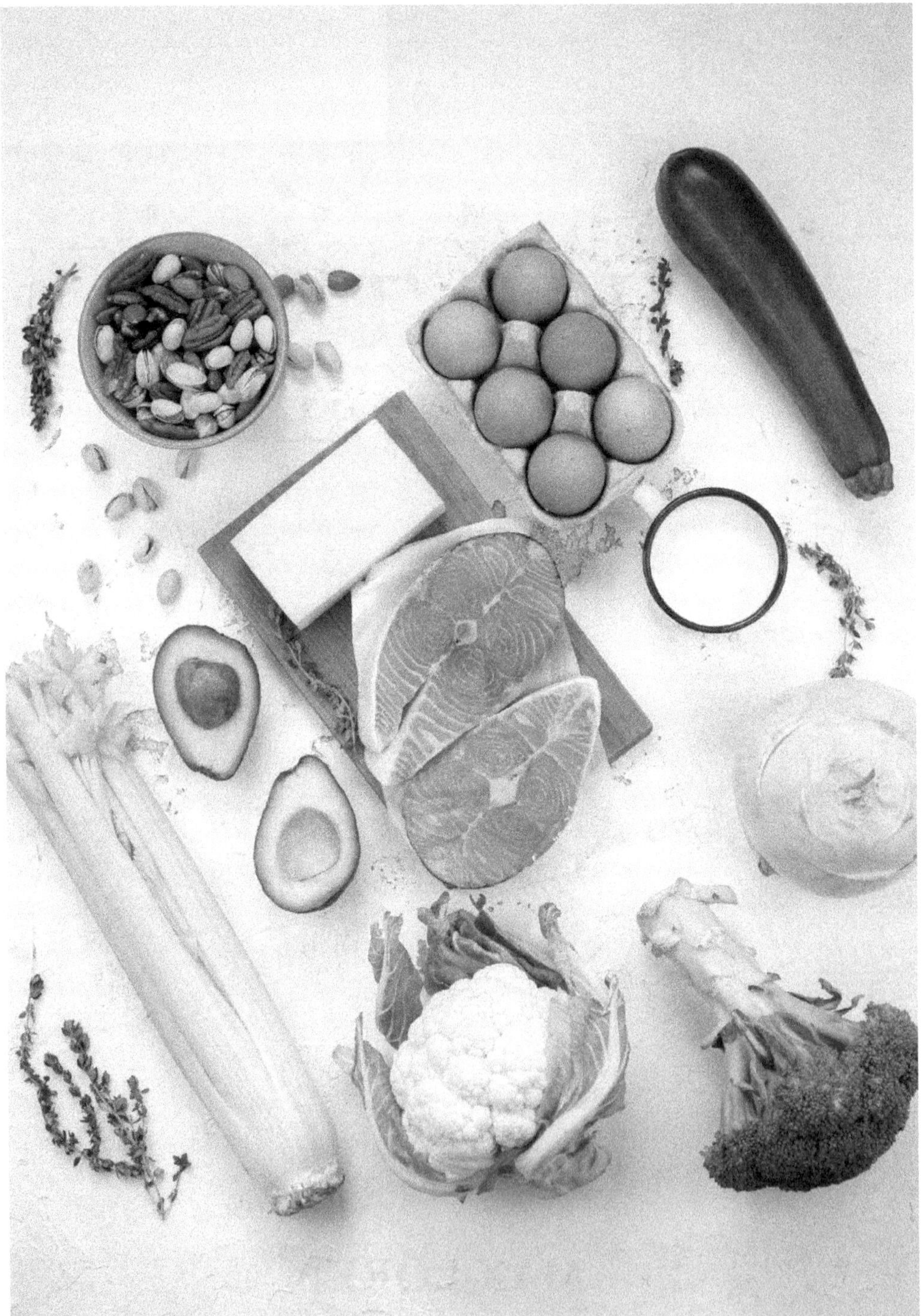

Legal Notice:

Disclaimer Notice:

Table of Contents

Sommario

Introduction

The ketogenic diet, or keto diet, is a low-carbohydrate, high-fat diet that provides many health benefits.Many studies have shown that this type of diet can help you reduce and improve your health.Ketogenic diets may even have benefits against diabetes, cancer, epilepsy, and Alzheimer's disease.

What is a ketogenic diet?

The ketogenic diet is a low carbohydrate, high-fat diet that has many similarities to the Atkins and low carb diets.It involves drastically reducing carbohydrate intake and replacing carbohydrates with fat. This drastic reduction in carbs puts your body into a metabolic state called ketosis.When this occurs, your body is incredibly efficient at burning fat for energy. It also converts fat into ketones within the liver, which can form the energy for the brain.Ketogenic diets can cause major reductions in blood glucose and insulin levels. This, along with the increase in ketones, has health benefits.

Different types of ketogenic diets

There are several versions of the ketogenic diet, including:

The standard ketogenic diet (SKD): This is often a low carb, moderate protein, and high-fat diet. It typically contains 70% fat, 20% protein, and only 10% carbs (9Trusted Source).

The cyclical ketogenic diet (CKD): This diet involves periods of upper carb refeeds, like 5 ketogenic days followed by 2 high carb days.

The targeted ketogenic diet (TKD): This diet allows you to feature carbs around workouts.

High protein ketogenic diet: this is often almost like a typical ketogenic diet, but includes more protein. The ratio is usually 60% fat, 35% protein, and 5% carbs.

However, only the quality and high protein ketogenic diets are studied extensively. Cyclical or targeted ketogenic diets are more advanced methods and are primarily employed by bodybuilders or athletes.

What is ketosis?

Ketosis may be a metabolic state during which your body uses fat for fuel rather than carbs.

It occurs once you significantly reduce your consumption of carbohydrates, limiting your body's supply of glucose (sugar), which is that the main source of energy for the cells.

Following a ketogenic diet is that the best thanks to entering ketosis. Generally, this involves limiting carb consumption to around 20 to 50 grams per day and filling abreast of fats, like meat, fish, eggs, nuts, and healthy oils

It's also important to moderate your protein consumption, this is often because protein can be converted into glucose if consumed in high amounts, which can slow your transition into ketosis

Practicing intermittent fasting could also assist you to enter ketosis faster. There are many various sorts of intermittent fasting, but the foremost common method involves limiting food intake to around 8 hours per day and fasting for the remaining 16 hours

Blood, urine, and breath tests are available, which may help determine whether you've entered ketosis by measuring the number of ketones produced by your body.

Certain symptoms can also indicate that you've entered ketosis, including increased thirst, dry mouth, frequent urination, and decreased hunger or appetite

Ketogenic diets can help you lose weight

A ketogenic diet is also an effective solution for losing weight and decreasing risk factors for disease.

Research has shown that the ketogenic diet can be very effective for weight loss as a low-fat diet.

What's more, the diet is so rich that you can lose weight without needing to count calories or track your food intake.

An analysis of 13 studies revealed that following a low-carb ketogenic diet was slightly superior for long-term weight loss compared to a low-fat diet.

It also led to a reduction in diastolic blood pressure and triglyceride levels.

Other health benefits of keto

- The ketogenic diet originated as a method of treating neurological diseases such as epilepsy.

- Studies have now shown that this diet may have benefits for a wide variety of different health conditions:

- Heart disease. The ketogenic diet can help improve risk factors such as body fat, HDL (good) cholesterol levels, blood pressure, and blood sugar.

- Cancer. Diet is currently being explored as an adjunct treatment for cancer because it may help slow tumor growth.

- Alzheimer's disease. The keto diet may help reduce the symptoms of Alzheimer's disease and slow its progression.

- Epilepsy. Research has shown that the ketogenic diet can cause significant reductions in seizures in epileptic children.

- Parkinson's disease. Although more research is needed, one study found that the diet helped improve symptoms of Parkinson's disease.

- Polycystic ovary syndrome. The ketogenic diet may help reduce insulin levels, which may play a key role in polycystic ovary syndrome.

- Brain injury. Some research suggests that the diet may improve the outcomes of traumatic brain injuries.

However, keep in mind that research in many of these areas is far from conclusive.

Foods to avoid

Any food high in carbohydrates should be reduced.

Here is a list of foods that should be reduced or eliminated on a ketogenic diet:

sugary foods: soda, juice, smoothies, cake, ice cream, candy, etc.

grains or starches: wheat products, rice, pasta, cereals, etc.

fruits: all fruits, except small portions of berries such as strawberries

beans or legumes: peas, beans, lentils, chickpeas, etc.

root and tuber vegetables: potatoes, sweet potatoes, carrots, parsnips, etc.

low-fat or diet products: low-fat mayonnaise, salad dressings, and condiments

some condiments or sauces: barbecue sauce, honey mustard, teriyaki sauce, ketchup, etc.

unhealthy fats: processed vegetable oils, mayonnaise, etc.

alcohol: beer, wine, liquor, mixed drinks

sugar-free diet foods: sugar-free candy, syrups, puddings, sweeteners, desserts, etc.

Foods to eat

You should focus most of your meals on these foods:

meat: red meat, steak, ham, sausage, bacon, chicken, and turkey

fatty fish: salmon, trout, tuna, and mackerel

eggs: whole pastured eggs or omega-3s

butter and cream: grass-fed butter and heavy cream

cheese: non-processed cheeses such as cheddar, goat, cream, blue, or mozzarella cheese

nuts and seeds: almonds, walnuts, flaxseeds, pumpkin seeds, chia seeds, etc.

healthy oils: extra virgin olive oil, coconut oil, and avocado oil

avocado: whole avocado or freshly made guacamole

low carb vegetables: green vegetables, tomatoes, onions, peppers, etc.

seasonings: salt, pepper, herbs, and spices

It's best to base your diet primarily on whole, single-ingredient foods. Here's a list of 44 healthy low-carb foods.

Healthy keto snacks

In case you get the urge to eat between meals, here are some healthy, keto-approved snacks:

fatty meat or fish

cheese

a handful of nuts or seeds

keto sushi bites

olives

one or two hard-boiled or deviled eggs

keto-friendly snack bars

90 percent dark chocolate

whole Greek yogurt mixed with nut butter and cocoa powder

peppers and guacamole

strawberries and plain cottage cheese

celery with salsa and guacamole

beef jerky

smaller portions of leftover meals

fat bombs

Keto tips and tricks

Although starting the ketogenic diet can be difficult, there are several tips and tricks you can use to make it easier.

Start by familiarizing yourself with food labels and checking the grams of fat, carbohydrates, and fiber to determine how your favorite foods can fit into your diet.

Planning your meals can also be beneficial and can help you save extra time during the week.

Tips for eating out on a ketogenic diet

Many restaurant meals can be made keto-friendly.

Most restaurants offer some type of meat or fish dish. Order this food and replace any high-carb food with extra vegetables.

Egg meals are also a good option, such as an omelet or eggs and bacon. Another favorite meal is burgers without a bun. You could also replace the fries with veggies. Add extra avocado, cheese, bacon, or eggs.

In Mexican restaurants, you can enjoy any type of meat with extra cheese, guacamole, salsa, and sour cream.

For dessert, ask for a tray of mixed cheeses or berries with cream.

At least, in the beginning, it's crucial to eat until you're full and avoid cutting calories too much. Usually, a ketogenic diet involves weight loss without intentional calorie restriction.

In this Keto cookbook, you can organize your Keto diet with the different dishes you'll find for meals throughout the day. Enjoy!

Breakfast

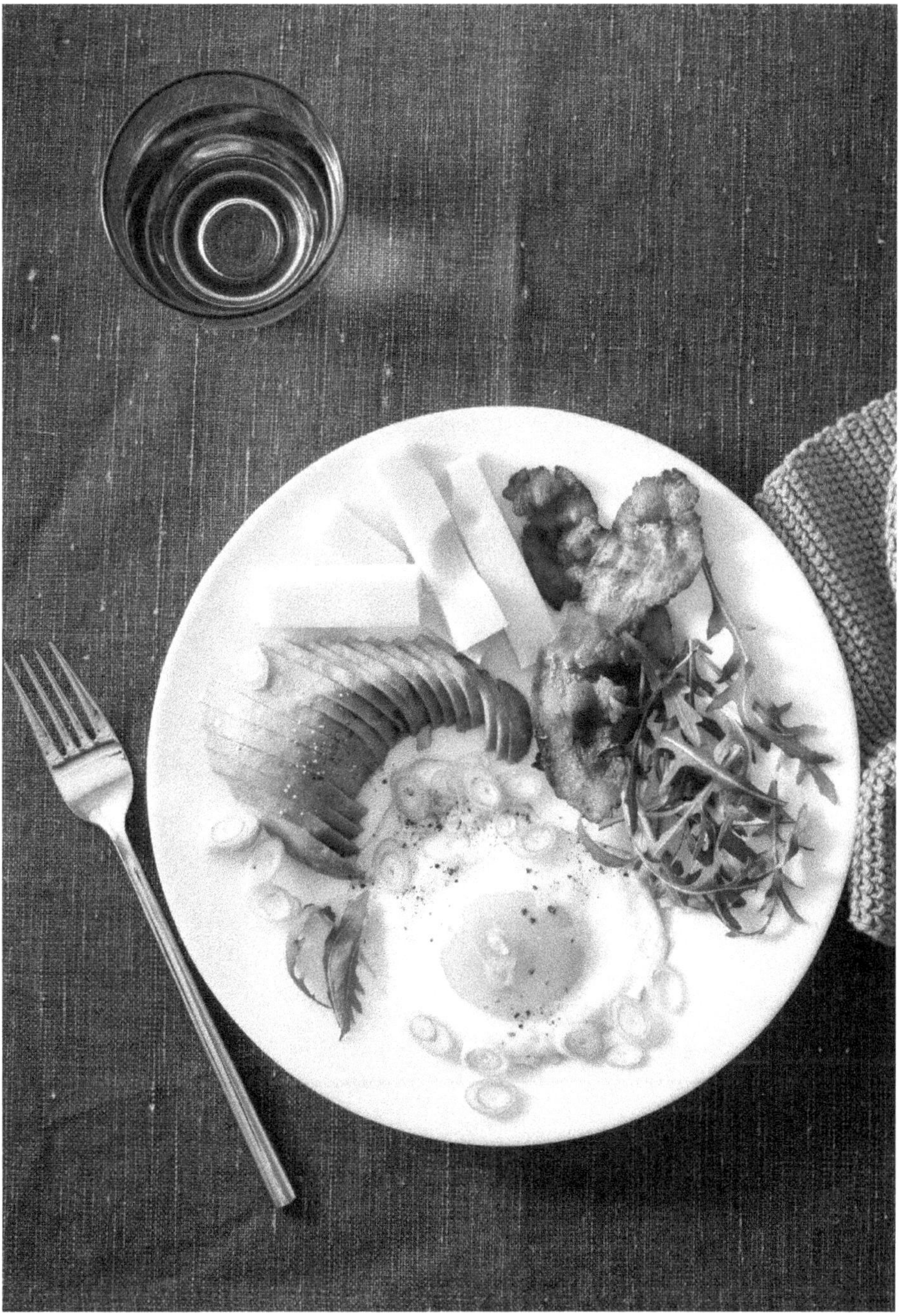

Cheesy Tater Tot Casserole

Preparation time: 10 minutes
Cooking time: 4 hours
Servings: 2

Ingredients:
Cooking spray
10 ounces tater tots, frozen
2 eggs, whisked
½ pound turkey sausage, ground
1 tablespoon heavy cream
¼ teaspoon thyme, dried
¼ teaspoon garlic powder
A pinch of salt and black pepper
½ cup Colby jack cheese, shredded

Directions:
Grease your slow cooker with cooking spray, spread tater tots on the bottom, add sausage, thyme, garlic powder, salt, pepper and whisked eggs.
Add cheese, cover pot and cook on Low for 4 hours.
Divide between plates and serve for breakfast.
Enjoy!

Nutrition:
Calories 231, Fat 5g, Fiber 9g, Carbs 15g, Protein 11g

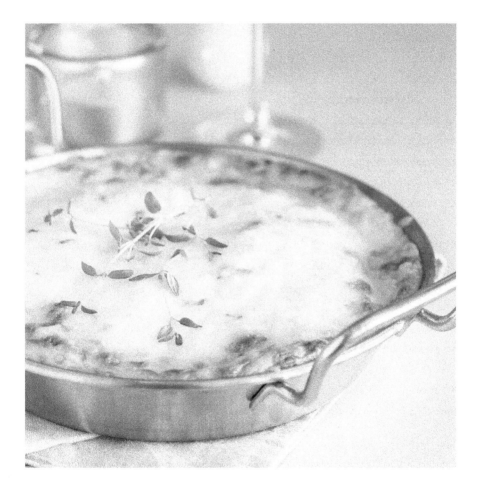

Apple Oatmeal

Preparation time: 20 minutes
Cooking time: 7 hours
Servings: 3

Ingredients:

¼ cup brown sugar

¼ teaspoon salt

2 cups milk

2 tablespoons honey

2 tablespoons butter, melted

½ teaspoon cinnamon

2 cup apple, peeled and chopped

½ cup walnuts, chopped

1 cup steel cut oats

½ cup dates, chopped

Directions:

Grease a crock pot and add milk, honey, brown sugar, melted butter, cinnamon and salt.

Mix well and stir in the oats, apples, walnuts and dates.

Cover and cook on LOW for about 7 hours.

Dish out and stir well before serving.

Nutrition:

calories 593, fat 25.3g, carbohydrates 84.8g

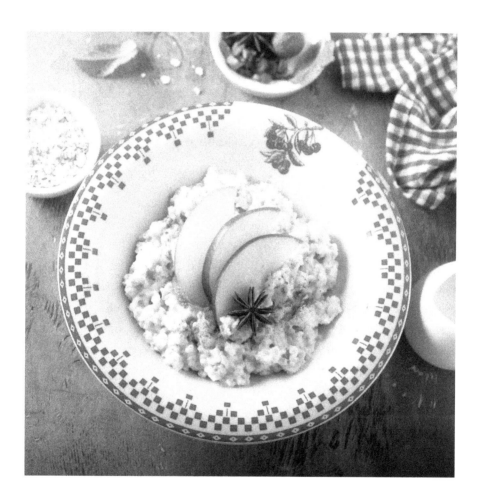

Green Vegetable Quiche

Preparation Time: 20 minutes
Cooking Time: 20 minutes
Servings: 4

Ingredients:
6 organic eggs
1/2 cup unsweetened almond milk
Salt and ground black pepper, as required
2 cups fresh baby spinach, chopped
1/2 cup green bell pepper, seeded and chopped
1 scallion, chopped
1/4 cup fresh cilantro, chopped
1 tablespoon fresh chives, minced
3 tablespoons mozzarella cheese, grated

Directions:
Preheat your oven to 400°F. Lightly grease a pie dish. In a bowl, add eggs, almond milk, salt, and black pepper, and beat until well combined. Set aside. In another bowl, add the vegetables and herbs and mix well. At the bottom of the prepared pie dish, place the veggie mixture evenly and top with the egg mixture. Let the quiche bake for about 20 minutes. Remove the pie dish from the oven and immediately sprinkle with the Parmesan cheese. Set aside for about 5 minutes before slicing. Cut into desired sized wedges and serve warm.

Nutrition:
calories 298, fat 10.4g, fiber 5.9g, carbohydrates 4.1 g, protein 7.9g

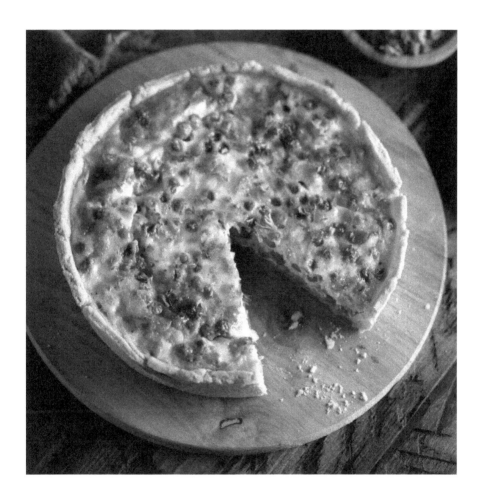

Ham Frittata

Preparation time: 10 minutes
Cooking time: 3 hours
Servings: 4

Ingredients:
4 eggs
10 oz ham, chopped
1 teaspoon butter
1 tablespoon dried dill
1 tablespoon dried parsley
¼ teaspoon salt
¾ cup almond milk, unsweetened

Directions:
Whisk the eggs in a mixing bowl with a hand whisker.
Add dried dill, chopped ham, dried parsley, salt, and almond milk.
Whisk the mixture well.
Add the butter to the slow cooker. Add egg mixture and close the lid.
Cook the frittata for 3 hours on Low.
Serve the cooked meal immediately!

Nutrition:
calories 283, fat 22.2g, fiber 2.1g, carbs 5g, protein 18.5g

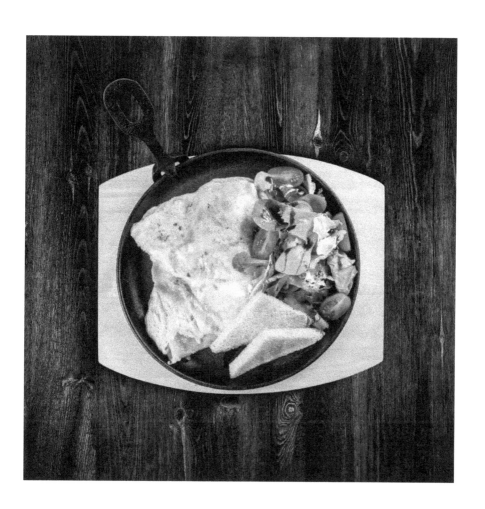

Pumpkin Oatmeal

Preparation time: 10 minutes
Cooking time: 7 hours
Servings: 2

Ingredients:
Cooking spray
½ cup steel cut oats
1 cup water
1 cup almond milk
1 and ½ tablespoon maple syrup
½ teaspoon vanilla extract
½ teaspoon pumpkin pie spice
½ cup pumpkin, chopped
¼ teaspoon cinnamon powder

Directions:
Grease your slow cooker with cooking spray, add steel cut oats, water, almond milk, maple syrup, vanilla, pumpkin spice, pumpkin and cinnamon, stir, cover and cook on Low for 7 hours.
Stir one more time, divide into bowls and serve.
Enjoy!

Nutrition:
Calories 242, fat 3g, fiber 8g, carbs 20g, protein 7g

Breakfast Tender Chicken Strips

Preparation time: 5 hours
Servings: 5

Ingredients:
1-pound chicken fillets
tablespoons butter
1 teaspoon dried dill
1 teaspoon dried oregano
teaspoon dried parsley
tablespoons full-fat cream

Directions:
Cut the chicken fillets into the strips.
Then sprinkle the chicken strips with the dried dill, oregano, and parsley.
Toss the poultry with the full-fat cream.
Place the butter in the slow cooker and add the chicken strips.
Then close the lid and cook the chicken strips for 5 hours on Low.
Stir the cooked chicken strips and transfer onto a serving platter.
Enjoy!

Nutrition:
calories 222, fat 12.1g, fiber 0.2g, carbs 0.6g, protein 26.6g

Chai Waffles

Preparation Time: 15 minutes
Cooking Time: 20 minutes
Servings: 4

Ingredients:
4 eggs, separated
3 tablespoons coconut flour
3 tablespoons powdered Erythritol
1 1/4 teaspoon baking powder
1 teaspoon vanilla extract
1/2 teaspoon ground cinnamon
1/4 teaspoon ground ginger
Pinch ground cloves
Pinch ground cardamom
3 tablespoons coconut oil, melted
3 tablespoons unsweetened almond milk

Directions:
Divide the eggs into two separate mixing bowls. Whip the whites until stiff peaks develop and then set aside. Whisk the egg yolks into the other bowl with the coconut flour, Erythritol, baking powder, cocoa, cinnamon, cardamom, and cloves. Pour the melted coconut oil and the almond milk into the second bowl and whisk. Fold softly in the whites of the egg until you have just combined. Preheat waffle iron with cooking spray and grease. Spoon into the iron for about 1/2 cup of batter. Cook the waffle according to directions from the maker. Move the waffle to a plate and repeat with the batter leftover.

Nutrition:
calories 286, fat 13.9g, fiber 8.5g, carbohydrates 4.8 g, protein 12.8 g

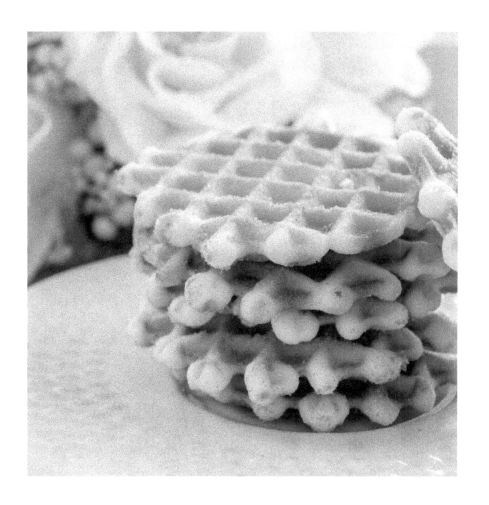

Chicken

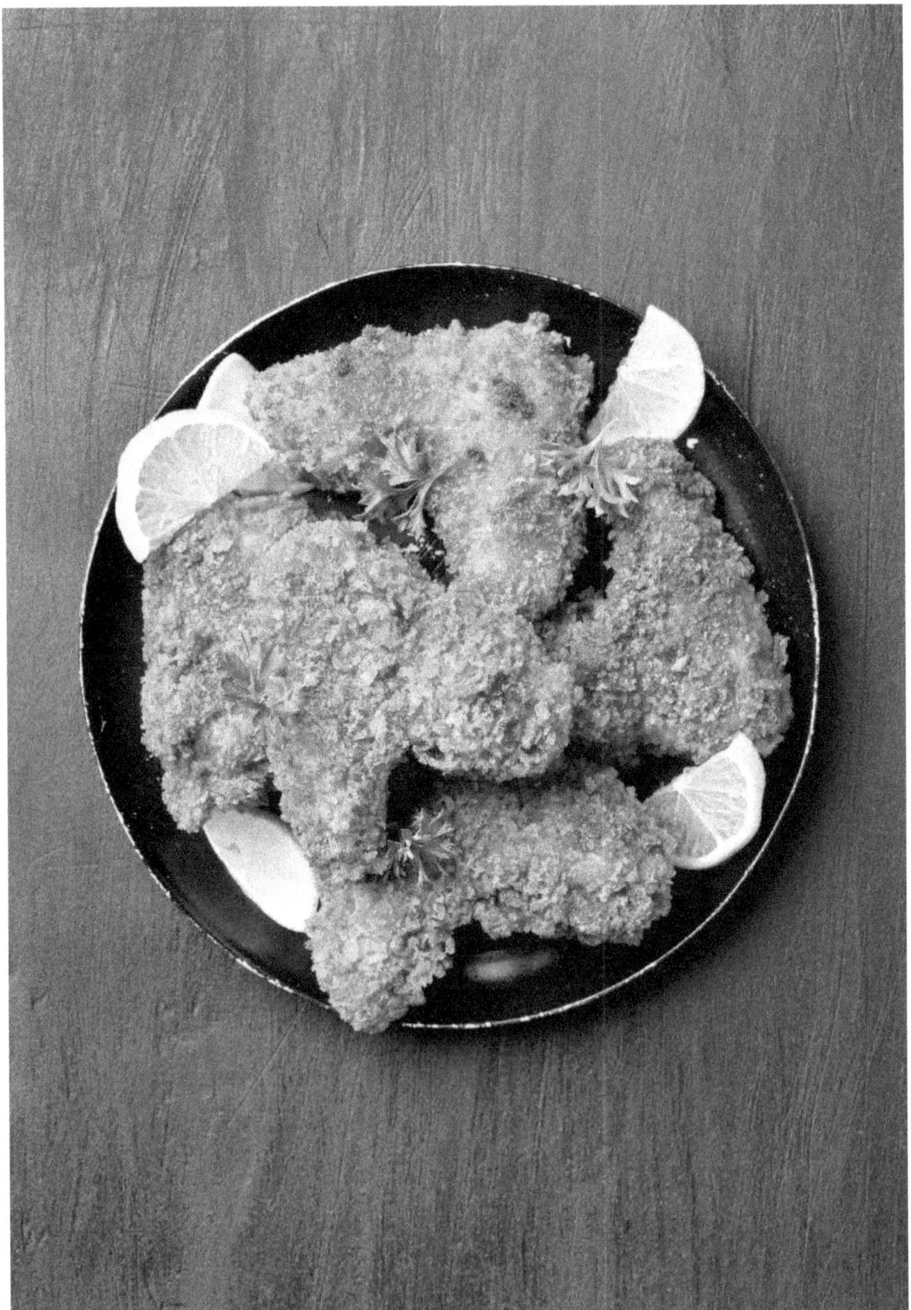

Turkey Meatballs

Preparation Time: 15 minutes
Cooking Time: 20 minutes
Servings: 2

Ingredients:

1 pound of ground turkey
1 tablespoon of fish sauce
diced onion
tablespoons of soy sauce
1/2 almond flour
1/8 cup of ground beef
1/2 teaspoon of garlic powder
1/2 teaspoon of salt
1/2 teaspoon of ground ginger
1/2 teaspoon of thyme
1/2 teaspoon of curry
5 tablespoons of olive oil

Directions:

Combine ground turkey, fish sauce, one diced onion, soy sauce, ground beef, seasonings, oil, and flour in a large mixing bowl. Mix it thoroughly.
Form meatballs depending on preferred size.
Heat skillet and pour in 3 tablespoons of oil [you may need more depending on the size of meat balls].
Cook meatballs until evenly browned on each side. Serve hot.

Nutrition:

calories 281, fat 11.6g, fiber 6.9g, carbohydrates 4.6g, protein 15.1g

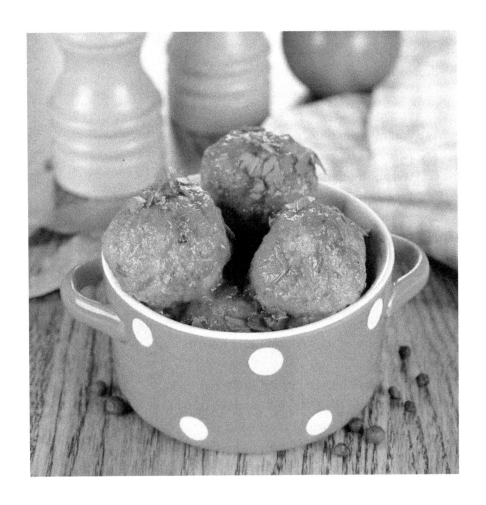

Mexican Cotija Chicken Breasts

Preparation time: 15 minutes
Cooking time: 20 minutes
Servings: 6

Ingredients:

2 tablespoons olive oil
1½ pounds (680 g) chicken breasts, cut into bite-sized cubes
1 teaspoon garlic, finely chopped
Mexican chili pepper, finely chopped
ripe tomatoes, puréed
Sea salt and black pepper, to taste
½ teaspoon paprika
½ teaspoon Mexican oregano
4 ounces (113 g) sour cream
6 ounces (170 g) Cotija cheese, crumbled
2 tablespoons fresh chives, chopped

Directions:

Heat the olive oil in a frying pan over a medium-high flame. Now, brown the chicken breasts for 4 to 5 minutes per side.

Then, sauté the garlic and pepper until they are tender and aromatic. Fold in the puréed tomatoes and cook for a further 4 minutes. Season with salt, black pepper, paprika, and Mexican oregano. Transfer the chicken with the sauce to a lightly greased casserole dish.

Top with the sour cream and Cotija cheese. Bake in the preheated oven for 12 to 13 minutes or until thoroughly cooked.

Garnish with fresh chives and serve warm.

Nutrition:

calories 355, fat 23.1g, protein 29.2g, carbs 5.9g, net carbs 5.4g, fiber 0.5g

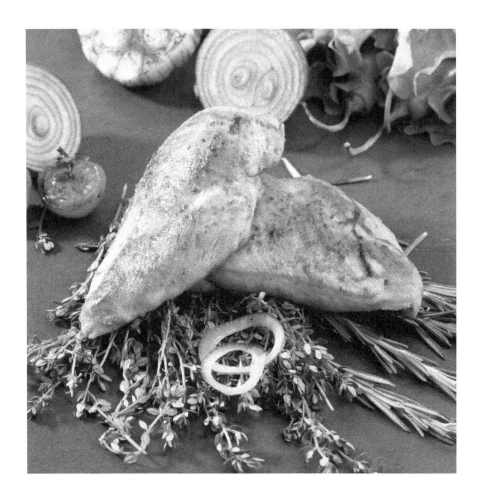

Chicken Quesadilla

Preparation Time: 15 minutes
Cooking Time: 25 minutes
Servings: 4

Ingredients:
1 tbsp. extra-virgin olive oil
1 bell pepper, sliced
1/2 yellow onion, sliced
1/2 tsp. chili powder
Kosher salt
Freshly ground black pepper 3
c. shredded Monterey Jack
c. shredded cheddar
c. shredded chicken
1 avocado, thinly sliced
1 green onion, thinly sliced
Sour cream, for serving

Directions:

Let the oven preheat to 400F. Prepare two baking sheets with a baking mat or parchment paper. Heat oil. Put pepper and onion and season with chili powder, salt, and pepper. Cook until soft, 5 minutes. Transfer to a plate. In a medium bowl, stir together cheeses. Put 1 1/2 cups of cheese mixture onto both prepared baking sheets centers. Spread the cheese evenly in a circle shape, like a flour tortilla. Bake the quesadilla for about 20 minutes. Put onion-pepper mixture, shredded chicken, and avocado slices to one half of each. Let cool slightly. Then use the parchment paper and a little spatula to gently lift. Fold the cheese tortillas empty side over the filling side. Place the quesadilla baking sheet in the oven to heat, 3 to 5 minutes more. Decorate with green onion and sour cream and serve.

Nutrition:

calories 299, fat 12.1g, fiber 4.1g, carbohydrates 4.1g, protein 10.1

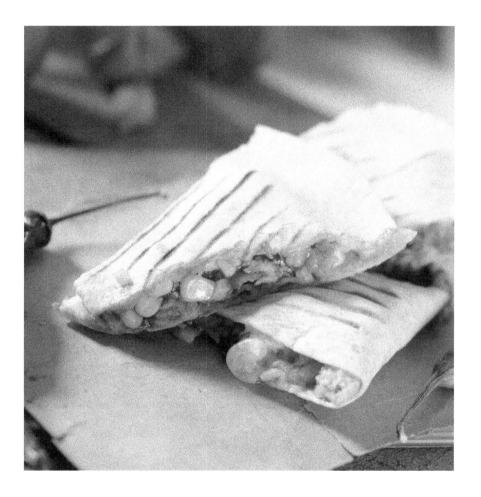

Chinese Flavor Chicken Legs

Preparation time: 10 minutes
Cooking time: 15 minutes
Servings: 4

Ingredients:
1 tablespoon sesame oil
4 chicken legs
¼ cup Shaoxing wine
2 tablespoons brown erythritol
¼ cup spicy tomato sauce

Directions:
Heat the sesame oil in a cast-iron skillet over medium-high flame. Now, sear chicken wings until they turn golden in color on all sides; reserve.

Then, in the same skillet, add a splash of wine to deglaze the pan.

Add in the remaining wine, brown erythritol, and spicy tomato sauce. Bring to a boil and immediately reduce the heat to medium-low.

Let it simmer for 5 to 10 minutes until the sauce coats the back of a spoon. Add the reserved chicken legs back to the skillet.

Cook for a further 3 minutes or until the chicken is well coated and heated through. Enjoy!

Nutrition:
calories 366, fat 14.6g, protein 51.1g, carbs 3.4g, net carbs 2.4g, fiber 1.0g

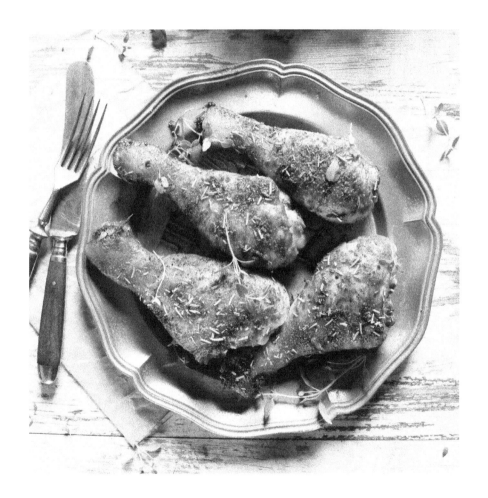

Leek and Pumpkin Turkey Stew

Preparation time: 20 minutes
Cooking time: 7 to 8 hours
Servings: 6

Ingredients:
3 tablespoons extra-virgin olive oil, divided
1 pound (454 g) boneless turkey breast, cut into 1-inch pieces
leek, thoroughly cleaned and sliced
teaspoons minced garlic
2 cups chicken broth
cup coconut milk
celery stalks, chopped
2 cups diced pumpkin
carrot, diced
teaspoons chopped thyme
Salt, for seasoning
Freshly ground black pepper, for seasoning
1 scallion, white and green parts, chopped, for garnish

Directions:
Lightly grease the insert of the slow cooker with 1 tablespoon of the
olive oil. In a large skillet over medium-high heat, heat the remaining 2
tablespoons of the olive oil. Add the turkey and sauté until browned,
about 5 minutes. Add the leek and garlic and sauté for an additional 3
minutes. Transfer the turkey mixture to the insert and stir in the broth,
coconut milk, celery, pumpkin, carrot, and thyme. Cover and cook on
low for 7 to 8 hours. Season with salt and pepper.
Serve topped with the scallion.

Nutrition:
calories 357, fat 27.0g, protein 21.0g, carbs 11.0g, net carbs 7.0g,
fiber 4.0g

Ranch Turkey with Greek Aioli Sauce

Preparation time: 10 minutes
Cooking time: 15 minutes
Servings: 4

Ingredients:
2 eggs
Kosher salt and ground black pepper, to taste
teaspoon paprika
tablespoons pork rinds
2 tablespoons flaxseed meal
½ cup almond meal
pound (454 g)turkey tenders, ½-inch thick
tablespoons sesame seeds
2 tablespoons olive oil
Sauce:
2 tablespoons Greek aioli
½ cup Greek yogurt
Flaky sea salt and freshly ground black pepper, to season

Directions:
In a mixing bowl, whisk the eggs with salt and black pepper until well combined. In a separate bowl, make the keto breading. Thoroughly combine the paprika, pork rinds, flaxseed meal, and almond meal. Dip the turkey tenders into the egg mixture. Then, press the turkey tenders into the keto breading. Dip them into the egg mixture again and roll them over the sesame seeds to coat well. Heat the olive oil in a large frying pan over medium-high heat. Once hot, add the turkey tenders and let them brown, about 4 minutes per side. Meanwhile, whisk the sauce ingredients until everything is well incorporated. Serve the turkey tenders with the sauce on the side. Enjoy!

Nutrition:
calories 397, fat 27.4g, protein 32.9g, carbs 3.8g, net carbs 2.0g, fiber 1.8g

Italian Turkey Meatballs with Leeks

Preparation time: 10 minutes
Cooking time: 20 minutes
Servings: 4

Ingredients:
1 pound (454 g) ground turkey
tablespoon Italian seasoning blend
cloves garlic, minced
½ cup leeks, minced
1 egg

Directions:
Throw all ingredients into a mixing bowl; mix to combine well.
Form the mixture into bite-sized balls and arrange them on a parchment-lined baking pan. Spritz the meatballs with cooking spray.
Bake in the preheated oven at 400°F (205°C) for 18 to 22 minutes. Serve with cocktail sticks and enjoy!

Nutrition:
calories 217, fat 11.1g, protein 24.1g, carbs 3.4g, net carbs 2.8g, fiber 0.6g

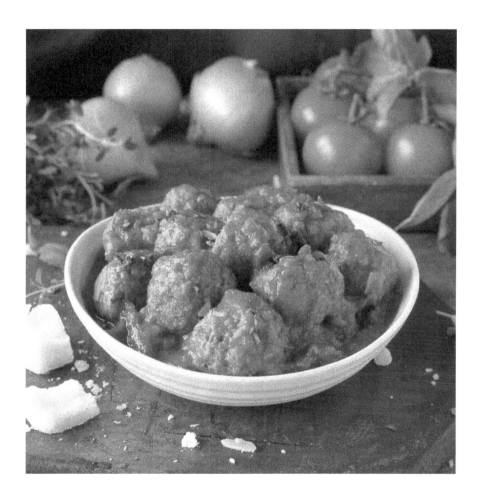

Pork

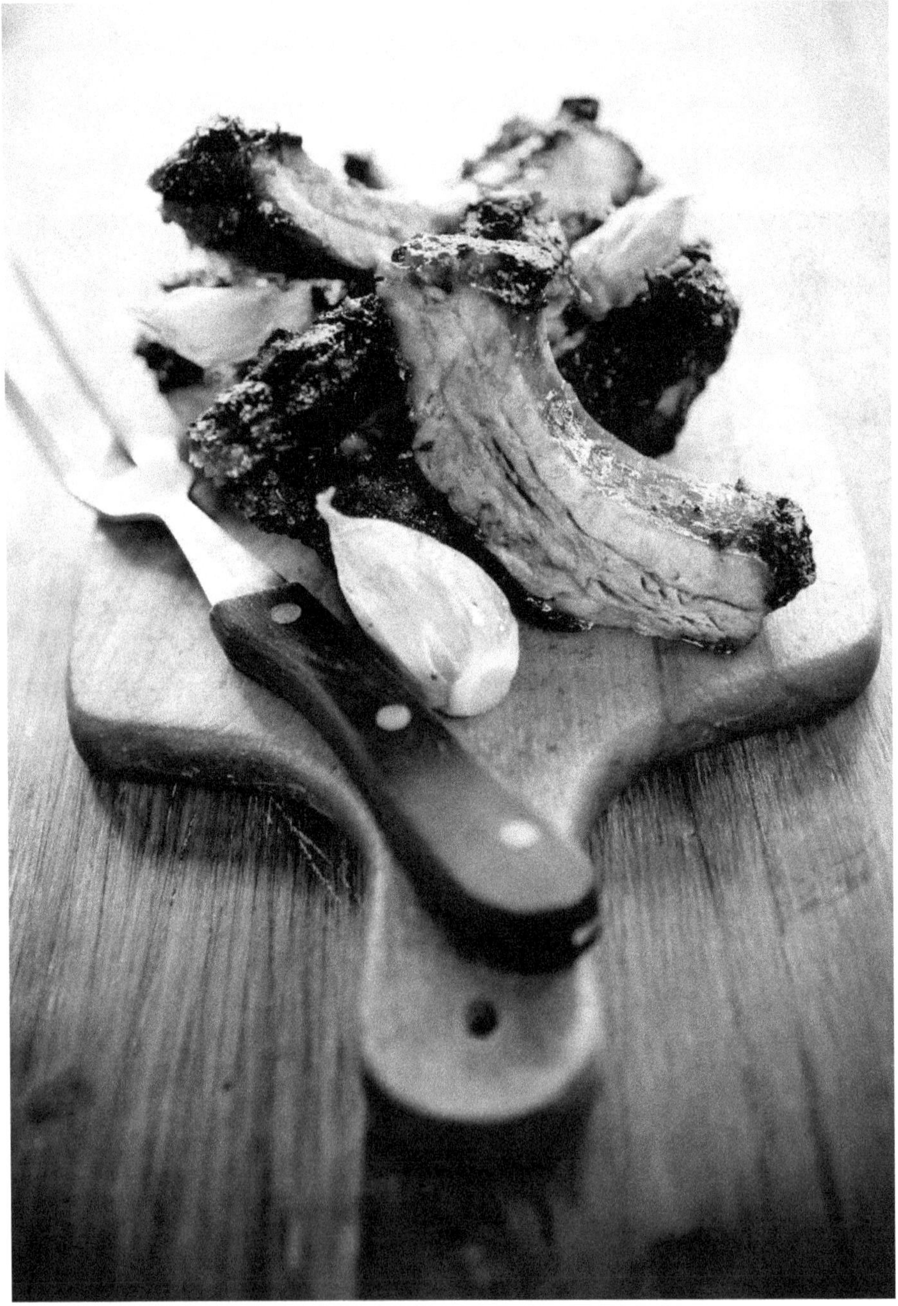

Coconut and Lime Steak

Preparation Time: 25 minutes
Cooking Time: 15 minutes
Servings: 4

Ingredients:
2 pounds steak, grass-fed
1 tablespoon minced garlic
1 lime, zested
1 teaspoon ginger, grated
3/4 teaspoon sea salt
teaspoon red pepper flakes
tablespoons lime juice
1/2 cup coconut oil, melted

Directions:
Take a large bowl and add garlic, ginger, salt, red pepper flakes, lime juice, zest, pour in oil, and whisk until combined.
Add the steaks, toss until well coated, and marinate at room temperature for 20 minutes.
After 20 minutes, take a large skillet pan, place it over medium-high heat, and when hot, add steaks (cut steaks in half if they don't fit into the pan).
Cook the steaks and then transfer them to a cutting board.
Let steaks cool for 5 minutes, then slice across the grain and serve.

Nutrition:
calories 512, fat 17.9g, fiber 12.5g, carbohydrates 4.9 g, protein 19.9g

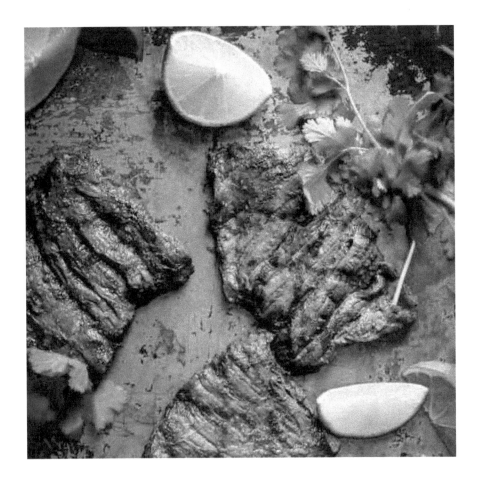

Spicy Tomato Pork Chops

Preparation time: 15 minutes
Cooking time: 36 minutes
Servings: 4

Ingredients:
4 pork chops
tablespoon fresh oregano, chopped
garlic cloves, minced1 tablespoon canola oil
15 ounces (425 g) canned diced tomatoes
1 tablespoon tomato paste
Salt and black pepper, to taste
¼ cup tomato juice
1 red chili, finely chopped

Directions:
Set a pan over medium heat and warm oil, place in the pork, season with pepper and salt, cook for 6 minutes on both sides; remove to a bowl. Add in the garlic, and cook for 30 seconds. Stir in the tomato paste, tomatoes, tomato juice, and chili; bring to a boil, and reduce heat to medium-low.
Place in the pork chops, cover the pan and simmer everything for 30 minutes. Remove the pork to plates and sprinkle with fresh oregano to serve.

Nutrition:
calories 412, fat 21.0g, protein 39.1g, carbs 6.3g, net carbs 3.5g, fiber 2.8g

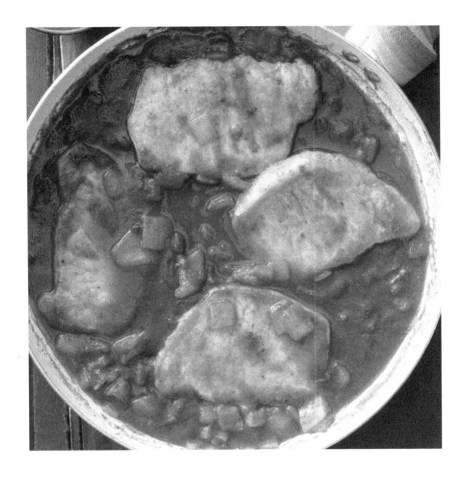

Mushroom and Pork Bake

Preparation time: 10 minutes
Cooking time: 45 minutes
Servings: 6

Ingredients:
onion, chopped
(10.5-ounce / 298-g) cans mushroom soup
6 pork chops
½ cup sliced mushrooms
Salt and ground pepper, to taste

Directions:
Preheat the oven to 370°F (188°C).
Season the pork chops with salt and black pepper, and place in a baking dish.
Combine the mushroom soup, mushrooms, and onion, in a bowl. Pour this mixture over the pork chops. Bake for 45 minutes.

Nutrition:
calories 402, fat 32.5g, protein 19.5g, carbs 8.4g, net carbs 7.9g, fiber 0.5g

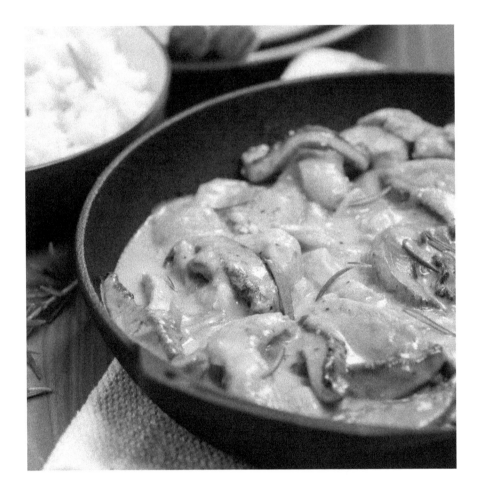

Pesto Pork Chops with Pistachios

Preparation time: 10 minutes
Cooking time: 2 hours
Servings: 4

Ingredients:

1 cup parsley
1 cup mint
1½ onions, chopped
⅓ cup pistachios
1 teaspoon lemon zest
5 tablespoons avocado oil
Salt, to taste
pork chops
garlic cloves, minced
Juice from 1 lemon

Directions:

In a food processor, combine the parsley with avocado oil, mint, pistachios, salt, lemon zest, and 1 onion. Rub the pork with this mixture, place in a bowl, and refrigerate for 1 hour while covered.
Remove the chops and set to a baking dish, place in ½ onion, and garlic; sprinkle with lemon juice, and bake for 2 hours in the oven at 250°F (121°C). Split amongst plates and enjoy.

Nutrition:

calories 565, fat 40.1g , protein 37.1g, carbs 8.3g, net carbs 5.4g, fiber 2.9g

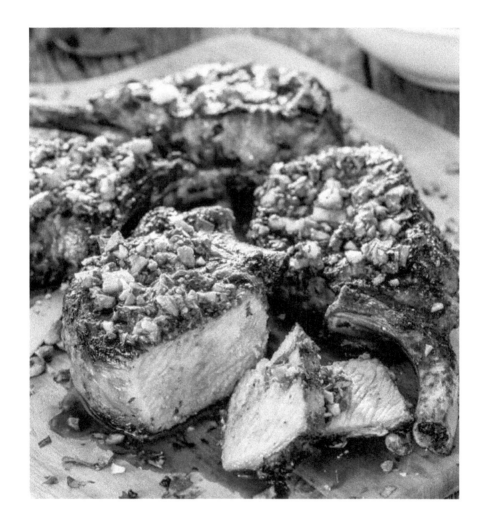

Cream of Onion Pork Cutlets

Preparation time: 10 minutes
Cooking time: 10 minutes
Servings: 4

Ingredients:
2 tablespoons olive oil
4 pork cutlets
¼ cup cream of onion soup
½ teaspoon paprika
Sea salt and ground black pepper, to taste

Directions:
Heat the olive oil in a sauté pan over moderate heat. Once hot, sear the pork cutlets for 5 to 6 minutes, turning once or twice to ensure even cooking.
Add in the cream of onion soup, paprika, salt, and black pepper. Cook for a further 3 minutes until heated through. The meat thermometer should register 145°F (63°C).
Serve in individual plates garnished with freshly snipped chives if desired. Enjoy!

Nutrition:
calories 396, fat 24.5g, protein 40.2g, carbs 0.9g, net carbs 0.7g, fiber 0.2g

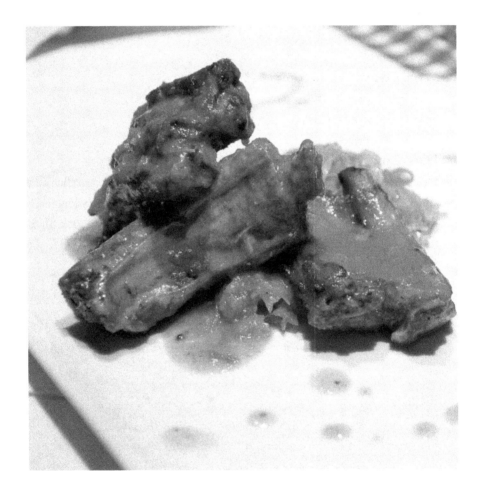

Texas Chili

Preparation time: 20 minutes
Cooking time: 7 to 8 hours
Servings: 4

Ingredients:

¼ cup extra-virgin olive oil
1½ pounds (680 g) beef sirloin, cut into 1-inch chunks
sweet onion, chopped
green bell peppers, chopped
jalapeño pepper, seeded, finely chopped
teaspoons minced garlic
1 (28-ounce / 794-g) can diced tomatoes
1 cup beef broth
3 tablespoons chili powder
½ teaspoon ground cumin
¼ teaspoon ground coriander
1 cup sour cream, for garnish
1 avocado, diced, for garnish
1 tablespoon cilantro, chopped, for garnish

Directions:

Lightly grease the insert of the slow cooker with 1 tablespoon of the olive oil. In a large skillet over medium-high heat, heat the remaining 2 tablespoons of the olive oil. Add the beef and sauté until it is cooked through, about 8 minutes. Add the onion, bell peppers, jalapeño pepper, and garlic, and sauté for an additional 4 minutes.
Transfer the beef mixture to the insert and stir in the tomatoes, broth, chili powder, cumin, and coriander. Cover and cook on low for 7 to 8 hours. Serve topped with the sour cream, avocado, and cilantro.

Nutrition:

calories 488, fat 38.1g, protein 25.9g. carbs 17.1g, net carbs 10.2g, fiber 6.9g

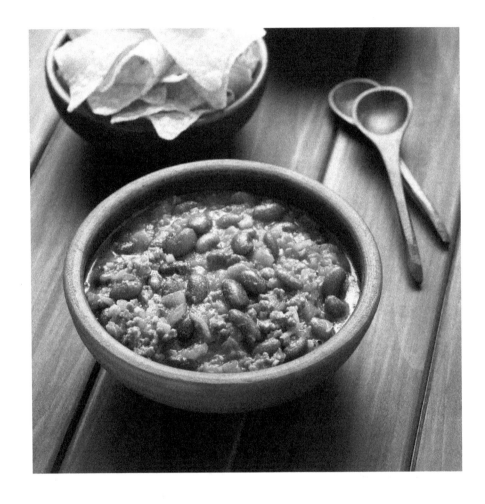

Pork Medallions

Preparation time: 15 minutes
Cooking time: 15 minutes
Servings: 2

Ingredients:
ounce (28 g) bacon, diced
pork medallions
2 garlic cloves, sliced
1 red onion, chopped
1 jalapeño pepper, deseeded and chopped
1 tablespoon apple cider vinegar
½ cup chicken bone broth
⅓ pound (136 g) red cabbage, shredded
1 bay leaf
1 sprig rosemary
1 sprig thyme
Kosher salt and ground black pepper, to taste

Directions:
Heat a Dutch pot over medium-high heat. Once hot, cook the bacon until it is crisp or about 3 minutes; reserve. Now, cook the pork medallions in the bacon grease until they are browned on both sides. Add the remaining ingredients and reduce the heat to medium-low. Let it cook for 13 minutes more, gently stirring periodically to ensure even cooking. Taste and adjust the seasonings. Serve in individual bowls topped with the reserved fried bacon. Bon appétit!

Nutrition:
calories 529, fat 31.7g, protein 51.1g, carbs 6.2g, net carbs 3.7g, fiber 2.5g

Fish and Seafood

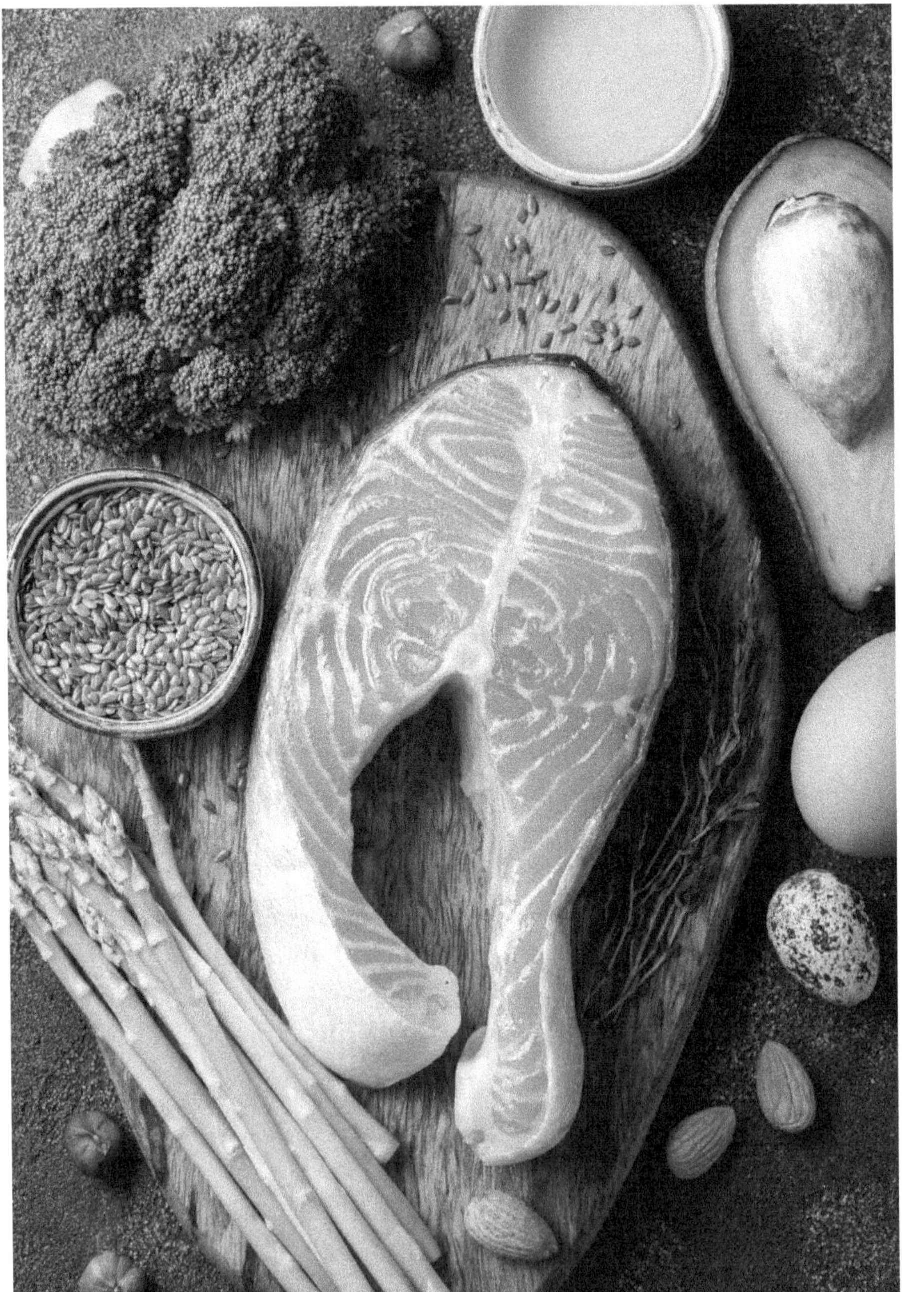

Coconut Crab Cakes

Preparation Time: 20 minutes
Cooking Time: 25 minutes
Servings: 4

Ingredients:
tablespoon of minced garlic
pasteurized eggs
2 teaspoons of coconut oil
3/4 cup of coconut flakes
3/4 cup chopped of spinach
1/4 pound crabmeat
1/4 cup of chopped leek
1/2 cup extra virgin olive oil
1/2 teaspoon of pepper
1/4 onion diced
Salt

Directions:
Pour the crabmeat in a bowl, then add in the coconut flakes and mix well.
Whisk eggs in a bowl, then mix in leek and spinach.
Season the egg mixture with pepper, two pinches of salt, and garlic.
Then, pour the eggs into the crab and stir well.
Preheat a pan, heat extra virgin olive, and fry the crab evenly from each side until golden brown.
Remove from pan and serve hot.

Nutrition:
calories 254, fat 9.5g, fiber 5.4g, carbohydrates 4.1 g, protein 8.9g

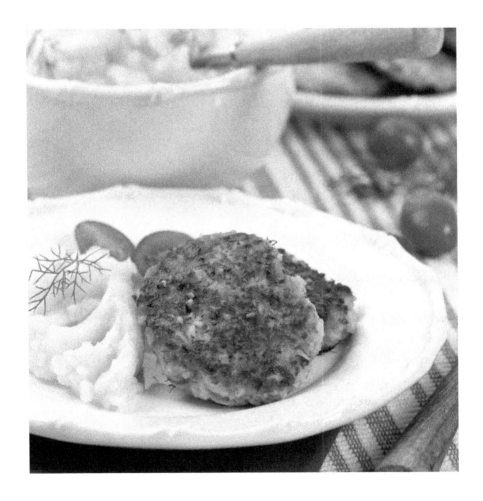

Seafood "Pasta"

Preparation time: 10 minutes
Cooking time: 6 hours
Servings: 6

Ingredients:
spaghetti squash (approximately 2 cups when cooked)
½ cup onion, sliced
½ cup red bell pepper, sliced
½ cup celery, diced
cloves garlic, crushed and minced
¼ cup butter, cubed
1 cup chicken or seafood stock
½ pound bay scallops
½ pound shrimp, cleaned and deveined
½ pound crab meat
½ cup heavy cream
½ cup goat cheese
1 tablespoon fresh tarragon
1 teaspoon salt
1 teaspoon black pepper

Directions:

Using a fork or sharp knife, poke 12-15 holes or small cuts in the surface of the spaghetti squash and place it in the center of the slow cooker. Add the onion, red bell pepper, celery, garlic, butter, and chicken or seafood stock around the squash. Cover and cook on high for 4 hours. Remove the lid of the slow cooker and remove the only the squash. Add the scallops, shrimp, crab meat, heavy cream, goat cheese, tarragon, salt and black pepper to the slow cooker. Toss gently. Cover the slow cooker and cook on high for an additional 15-20 minutes, or until all the seafood is cooked through. While the seafood is cooking, slice open the spaghetti squash and scoop out the contents. Transfer it to serving plates. Spoon the seafood and sauce over the spaghetti squash to serve.

Nutrition:

Calories 292.4, Fat 17.9g, Carbs 7.4g, Protein 25.2g, Fiber 1.3g, Sugars 2g

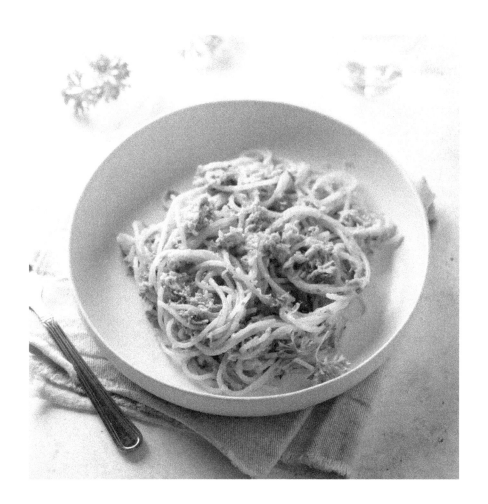

Orange Cod

Preparation time: 10 minutes
Cooking time: 3 hours
Servings: 4

Ingredients:
1-pound cod fillet, chopped
2 oranges, chopped
1 tablespoon maple syrup
1 cup of water
1 garlic clove, diced
1 teaspoon ground black pepper

Directions:
Mix cod with ground black pepper and transfer in the slow cooker.
Add garlic, water, maple syrup, and oranges.
Close the lid and cook the meal on High for 3 hours

Nutrition:
150 calories, 21.2g protein,, 14.8g carbohydrates, 1.2g fat, 2.4g fiber, 56mg cholesterol, 73mg sodium, 187mg potassium.

Scalloped Potatoes with Salmon

Preparation time: 10 minutes
Cooking time: 8 hours
Servings: 4

Ingredients:

3 tablespoons all-purposed flour
1 10¾-ounce can of cream of mushroom soup
5 medium-sized potatoes, peeled, and sliced
1 16-ounce can of salmon, drained and flaked
½ cup chopped onions
¼ cup water
Salt and pepper
Cooking spray

Directions:

Generously spray the slow cooker bottom and sides with cooking spray.

Place half of the potatoes in slow cooker. Sprinkle with half of the flour, then season with salt and pepper. Cover with half the flaked salmon, then sprinkle with half the onions. Repeat layers. Combine soup and water. Pour over top of potato and salmon mixture. Cover and cook on LOW for 7-8 hours or until potatoes are tender.

Nutrition:

calories 367, fat 22g, carbs 5.2g, protein 39g, sodium 849mg

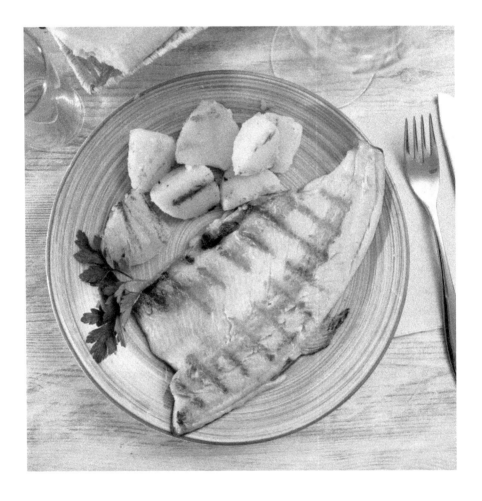

Miso Cod

Preparation time: 10 minutes
Cooking time: 4 hours
Servings: 4

Ingredients:
1-pound cod fillet, sliced
teaspoon miso paste
½ teaspoon ground ginger
cups chicken stock
½ teaspoon ground nutmeg

Directions:
In the mixing bowl mix chicken stock, ground nutmeg, ground ginger, and miso paste.
Then pour the liquid in the slow cooker.
Add cod fillet and close the lid.
Cook the fish on Low for 4 hours.

Nutrition:
101 calories, 20.8g protein, 1.1g carbohydrates, 1.5g fat, 0.2g fiber, 56mg cholesterol, 506mg sodium, 14mg potassium.

San Francisco Seafood Stew

Preparation time: 10 minutes
Cooking time: 5 hours
Servings: 8

Ingredients:
28-ounce can diced tomatoes, untrained
medium onions, chopped
celery stalks, chopped
1 8-ounce bottle clam juice
1 6-ounce can tomato paste
½ cup white wine (or vegetable broth)
5 cloves garlic, minced
1 tablespoon red wine vinegar
tablespoon olive oil
teaspoons Italian seasoning
1 bay leaf
½ teaspoon sugar
1 pound haddock fillets, cut into 1-inch pieces
1 pound shrimp (41-50 pieces per pound), uncooked, peeled and
deveined 1 6-ounce can chopped clams, undrained
6-ounce can lump crabmeat, drained
tablespoons minced fresh parsley

Directions:
Place the tomatoes, onions, celery, clam juice, tomato paste, wine or
broth, garlic, vinegar, olive oil, Italian seasoning, bay leaf, and sugar in a
slow cooker. Cover and cook 4-5 hours on LOW. Add the haddock,
shrimp, clams, and crabmeat. Cover and cook 20-30 minutes longer.
The soup is ready when the fish can easily be flaked and shrimp are
pink in color. Remove bay leaf. Stir in parsley and serve.

Nutrition:
Calories 205, Fat 3g, Carbs 15g, Protein 29g, Sodium 483mg

Macadamia Tilapia

Preparation time: 5 minutes
Cooking time: 15 minutes
Servings: 2

Ingredients:
2 (4-ounce / 113-g) tilapia fillets
½ cup unsalted macadamia nuts
1 tablespoon chopped fresh parsley
tablespoon fresh lemon juice
teaspoons coconut oil
¼ teaspoon garlic powder
Lemon wedges, for serving

Directions:
Preheat the oven to 400°F (205°C). Line a rimmed baking sheet with parchment paper.

Rinse the tilapia with cold water, pat dry with a paper towel, and place on the lined baking sheet.

Place the macadamia nuts, parsley, and lemon juice in a food processor and pulse/chop until the mixture is slightly chunkier than breadcrumb consistency. Be sure not to overblend, or you will end up with nut butter.

Top each fillet with 1 teaspoon of the coconut oil and then macadamia nut mixture, pressing it into the fish. Bake for 10 to 15 minutes, until the top is crisp and slightly golden brown. Serve with lemon wedges on the side.

Nutrition:
calories 82, fat 32.6g, protein 22.6g, carbs 5.4g, net carbs 2.6g, fiber 2.8g

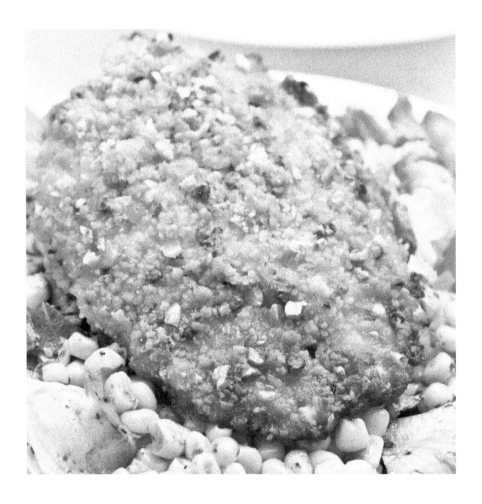

Soup

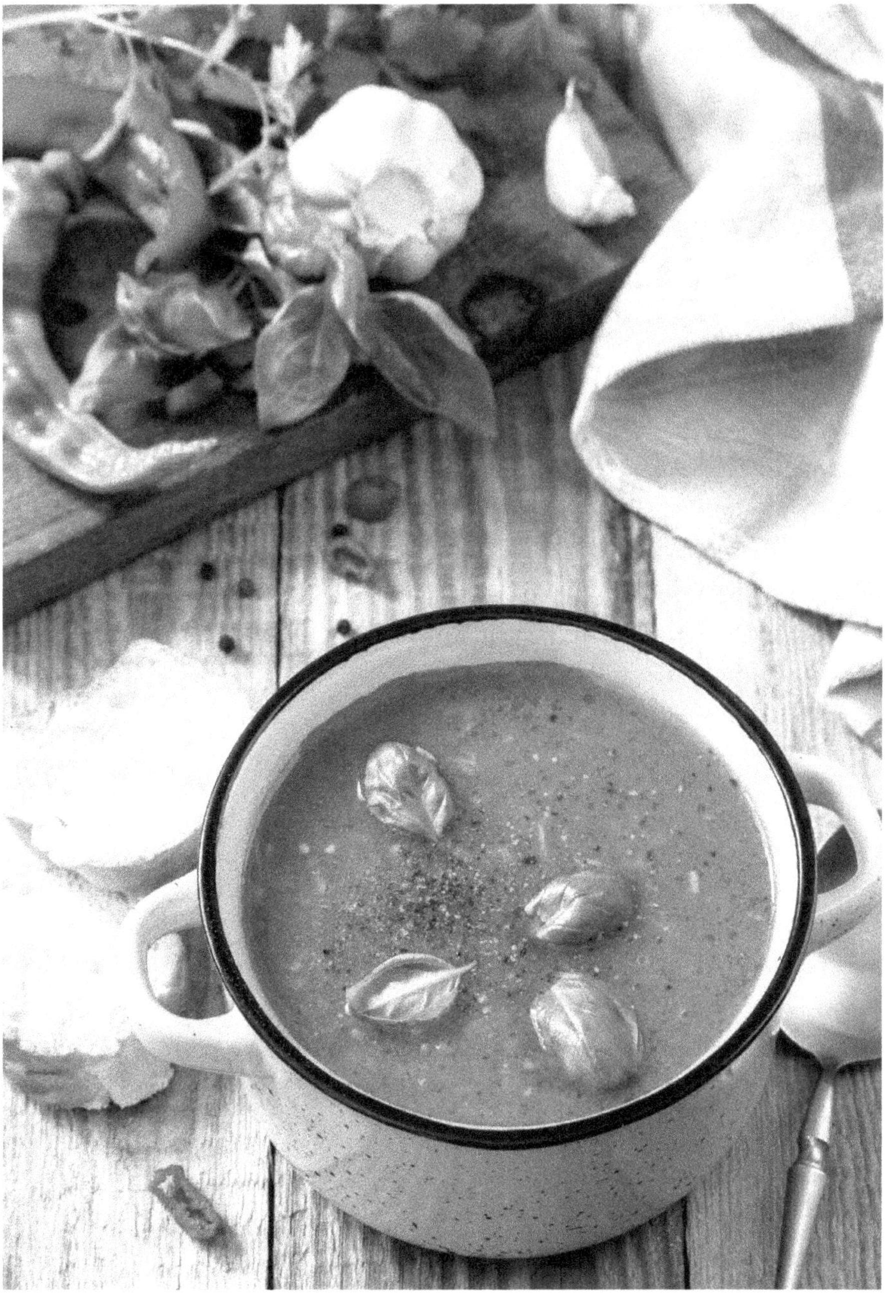

Leek and Turkey Soup

Preparation time: 15 minutes
Cooking time: 1 hour 10 minutes
Servings: 2

Ingredients:

3 cups water
½ pound (227 g) turkey thighs
1 cup cauliflower, broken into small florets
1 large-sized leek, chopped
1 small-sized stalk celery, chopped
½ head garlic, split horizontally
¼ teaspoon turmeric powder
¼ teaspoon Turkish sumac
¼ teaspoon fennel seeds
½ teaspoon mustard seeds
1 bay laurel
Sea salt and freshly ground black pepper, to season
1 teaspoon coconut aminos
1 whole egg

Directions:

Add the water and turkey thighs to a pot and bring it to a rolling boil. Cook for about 40 minutes; discard the bones and shred the meat using two forks.
Stir in the cauliflower, leeks, celery, garlic, and spices. Reduce the heat to simmer and let it cook until everything is heated through, about 30 minutes.
Afterwards, add the coconut aminos and egg; whisk until the egg is well incorporated into the soup. Serve hot and enjoy!

Nutrition:

calories 217, fat 8.2g, protein 25.1g, carbs 6.7g, net carbs 4.5g, fiber 2.2g

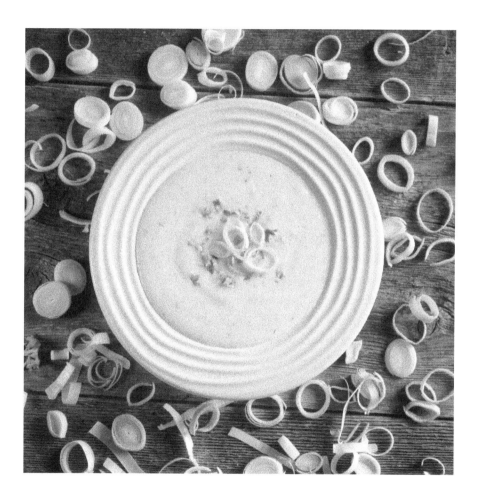

White Mushroom Soup

Preparation time: 15 minutes
Cooking time: 8 hours
Servings: 6

Ingredients:
9 oz. white mushrooms, chopped
6 chicken stock
1 teaspoon dried cilantro
½ teaspoon ground black pepper
1 teaspoon butter
1 cup potatoes, chopped
½ carrot, diced

Directions:
Melt butter in the skillet.
Add white mushrooms and roast them for 5 minutes on high heat. Stir the mushrooms constantly.
Transfer them in the slow cooker.
Add chicken stock, cilantro, ground black pepper, and potato.
Add carrot and close the lid.
Cook the soup on low for 8 hours.

Nutrition:
44 calories, 2.5g protein, 6.7g carbohydrates, 1.4g fat, 1.2g fiber, 2mg cholesterol, 776mg sodium, 271mg potassium.

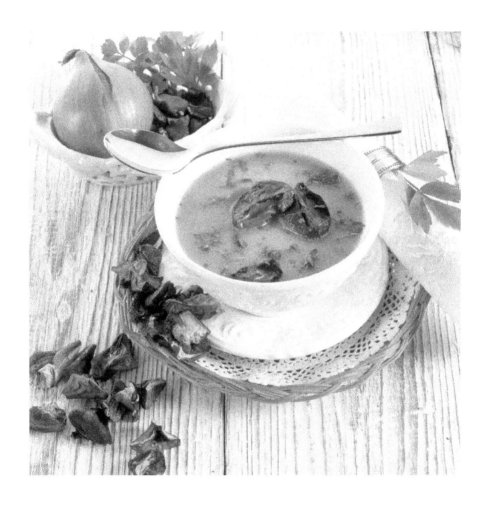

French Soup

Preparation time: 10 minutes
Cooking time: 7 hours
Servings: 5

Ingredients:
5 oz. Gruyere cheese, shredded
2 cups of water
2 cups chicken stock
2 cups white onion, diced
½ teaspoon cayenne pepper
½ cup heavy cream

Directions:
Pour chicken stock, water, and heavy cream in the slow cooker.
Add onion, cayenne pepper, and close the lid.
Cook the ingredients on high for 4 hours.
When the time is finished, open the lid, stir the mixture, and add cheese.
Carefully mix the soup and cook it on Low for 3 hours.

Nutrition:
181 calories, 9.5g protein, 5.1g carbohydrates, 13.9g fat, 1g fiber, 48mg cholesterol, 410mg sodium, 110mg potassium.

Hot Lentil Soup

Preparation time: 15 minutes
Cooking time: 24.5 hours
Servings: 4

Ingredients:
1 potato, peeled, diced
1 cup lentils
5 cups chicken stock
1 onion, diced
1 teaspoon chili powder
1 teaspoon cayenne pepper
1 teaspoon olive oil
1 tablespoon tomato paste

Directions:
Roast the onion in the olive oil until light brown and transfer in the slow cooker.
Add lentils, chicken stock, potato, chili powder, cayenne pepper, and tomato paste.
Carefully stir the soup mixture until the tomato paste is dissolved.
Close the lid and cook the soup on High for 4.5 hours.

Nutrition:
242 calories, 14.7g protein, 41.1g carbohydrates, 2.7g fat,
16.7g fiber, 0mg cholesterol, 972mg sodium, 758mg potassium.

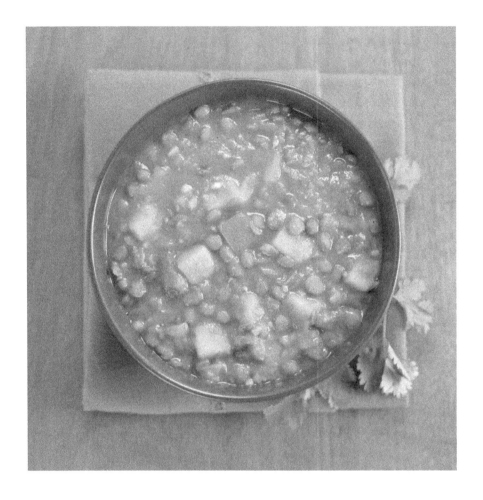

Cold Green Beans and Avocado Soup

Preparation Time: 15 minutes
Cooking Time: 15 minutes
Servings: 4

Ingredients:
tbsp. butter
tbsp. almond oil
1 garlic clove, minced
1 cup (227 g) green beans (fresh or frozen)
1/4 avocado
1 cup heavy cream
1/2 cup grated cheddar cheese + extra for garnish
1/2 tsp. coconut aminos
Salt to taste

Directions:
Heat the butter and almond oil in a large skillet and sauté the garlic for 30 seconds.
Add the green beans and stir-fry for 10 minutes or until tender. Add the mixture to a food processor and top with the avocado, heavy cream, cheddar cheese, coconut aminos, and salt. Blend the ingredients until smooth. Pour the soup into serving bowls, cover with plastic wraps and chill in the fridge for at least 2 hours. Enjoy afterward with a garnish of grated white sharp cheddar cheese

Nutrition:
calories 301, fat 3.1g, fiber 11.5g, carbohydrates 2.8 g, protein 3.1g

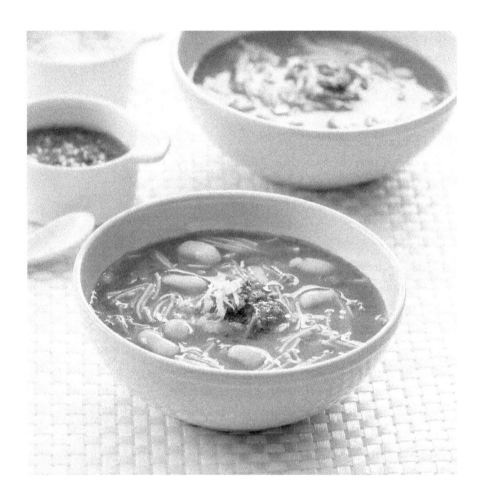

Sausage & Cheese Beer Soup

Preparation Time: 15 minutes
Cooking Time: 8 hrs.
Servings: 4

Ingredients:

2 tbsp. butter
1/2 cup celery, chopped
1/2 cup heavy cream
5 oz turkey sausage, sliced
small carrot, chopped
garlic cloves, minced
4 ounces cream cheese
1/2 tsp. red pepper flakes
1 cup beer of choice
3 cups beef stock
1 yellow onion, diced
1 cup cheddar cheese, grated
Kosher salt and black pepper, to taste
Fresh parsley, chopped, to garnish

Directions:

To the crockpot, add butter, beef stock, beer, turkey sausage, carrot, onion, garlic, celery, salt, red pepper flakes, and black pepper, and stir to combine.
Cook for 6 hrs. on low.
Then add in the cream, cheddar, and cream cheese, and cook for two more hours.

Nutrition:

calories 345, fat 10.4g, fiber 9.4g, carbohydrates 4.1 g, protein 11.2g

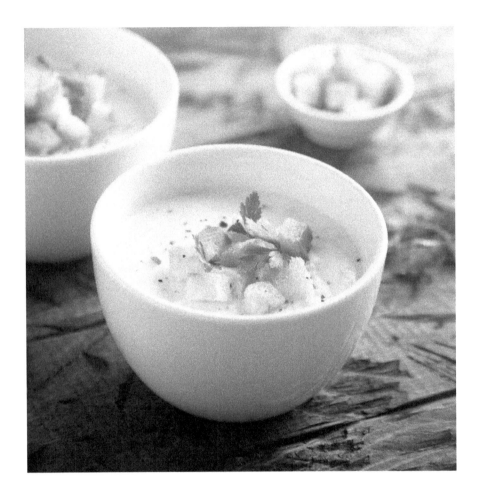

Chicken and Cauliflower Soup

Preparation time: 15 minutes
Cooking time: 7 to 8 hours
Servings: 6

Ingredients:
1 tablespoon extra-virgin olive oil
4 cups chicken broth
2 cups coconut milk
2 cups diced chicken breast
½ sweet onion, chopped
2 celery stalks, chopped
carrot, diced
½ cup chopped cauliflower
teaspoons minced garlic
1 teaspoon chopped thyme
1 teaspoon chopped oregano
¼ teaspoon freshly ground black pepper
Lightly grease the insert of the slow cooker with the olive oil.

Directions:
Add the broth, coconut milk, chicken, onion, celery, carrot, cauliflower, garlic, thyme, oregano, and pepper.
Cover and cook on low for 7 to 8 hours.
Serve warm.

Nutrition:
calories 300, fat 24.9g, protein 13.8g, carbs 7.9g, net carbs 5.1g, fiber 2.8g

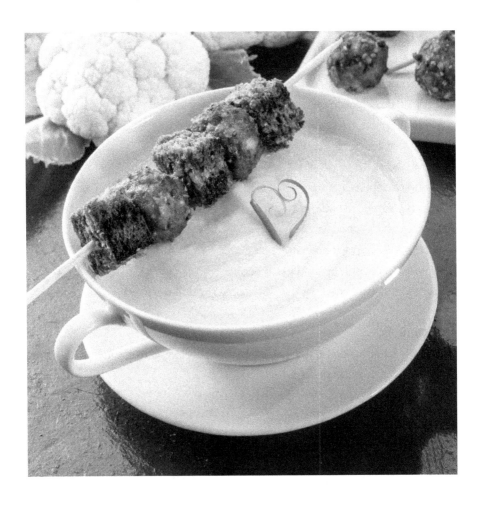

Snacks and Appetizer

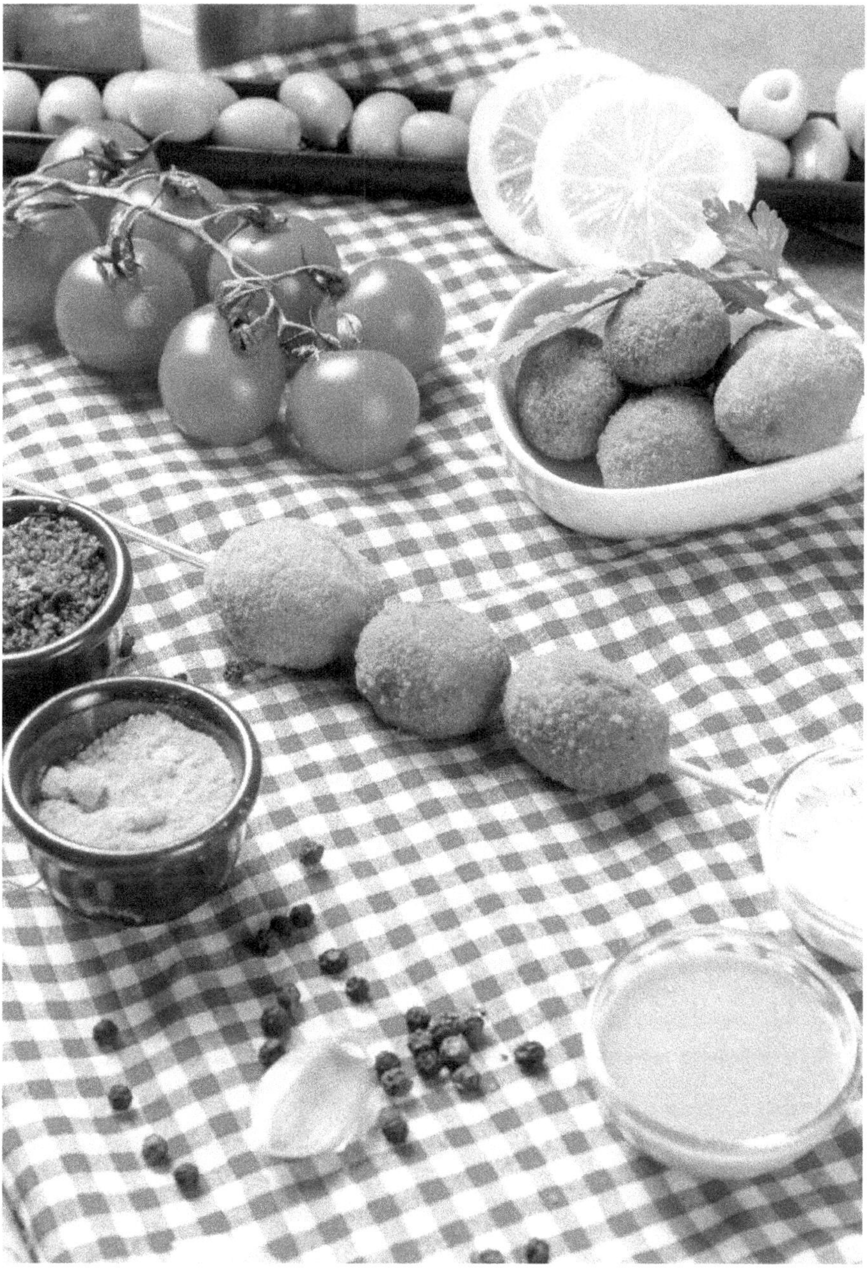

Zucchini Balls with Capers and Bacon

Preparation Time: 3 hrs.
Cooking Time: 20 minutes
Servings: 10

Ingredients:
2 zucchinis, shredded
2 bacon slices, chopped
1/2 cup cream cheese, at room temperature
1 cup fontina cheese
1/4 cup capers
1 clove garlic, crushed
1/2 cup grated Parmesan cheese
1/2 tsp. poppy seeds
1/4 tsp. dried dill weed
1/2 tsp. onion powder
Salt and black pepper, to taste
1 cup crushed pork rinds

Directions:
Preheat oven to 360 F.
Thoroughly mix zucchinis, capers, 1/2 of Parmesan cheese, garlic, cream cheese, bacon, and fontina cheese until well combined. Shape the mixture into balls. Refrigerate for 3 hours. In a mixing bowl, mix the remaining Parmesan cheese, crushed pork rinds, dill, black pepper, onion powder, poppy seeds, and salt. Roll cheese ball in Parmesan mixture to coat. Arrange in a greased baking dish in a single layer and bake in the oven for 15-20 minutes, shaking once.

Nutrition:
calories 227, fat 12.5g, fiber 9.4g, carbohydrates 4.3 g, protein 14.5g

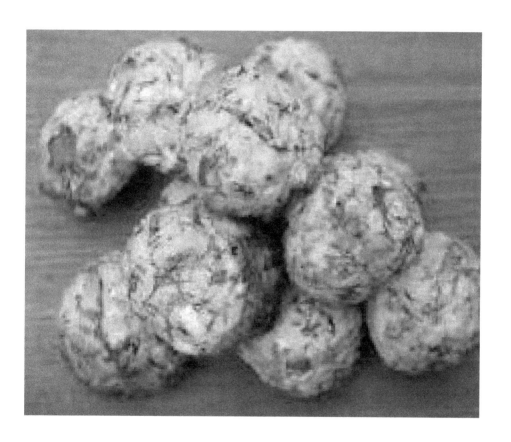

Tex Mex Dip

Preparation time: 10 minutes
Cooking time: 1 hour
Servings: 6

Ingredients:
15 ounces canned chili con carne
cup Mexican cheese, shredded
1 yellow onion, chopped
8 ounces cream cheese, cubed
½ cup beer
A pinch of salt
12 ounces macaroni, cooked
1 tablespoons cilantro, chopped

Directions:
In your slow cooker, mix chili con carne with cheese, onion, cream cheese, beer and salt, stir, cover and cook on High for 1 hour.
Add macaroni and cilantro, stir, divide into bowls and serve.

Nutrition:
calories 200, fat 4g, fiber 6g, carbs 17g, protein 5g

Marinated Mushrooms

Preparation time: 15 minutes
Cooking time: 3 hours
Servings: 8

Ingredients:
2 ounces dried mushrooms
2 (8-ounce) packages button mushrooms
2 tablespoons unsalted butter, plus more as needed
2 shallots, minced
¼ cup dry sherry (not cooking sherry)
1 tablespoon herbs de Provence
¼ teaspoon sea salt
¼ teaspoon freshly ground black pepper

Directions:
Place the dried mushrooms in a small bowl and cover with hot water. Let stand for 10 minutes to rehydrate. Drain; then remove the tough ends of the stems and discard. Coarsely chop the mushrooms and set aside. .Slice the larger fresh mushrooms in half, leaving the smaller ones whole. .Place a large skillet over high heat and melt the butter. Add half the button mushrooms and cook until browned; then push the first batch to the sides and add the remaining button mushrooms, adding more butter as needed to brown them. Transfer the browned mushrooms to a 3-quart slow cooker along with the chopped rehydrated dried mushrooms. In the same skillet, cook the shallots for about 3 minutes, or until slightly softened. Transfer the shallots to the slow cooker and add the sherry, herbes de Provence, salt, and pepper. Cover and cook on low for 2 to 3 hours, or until the button mushrooms are tender and brown.

Nutrition:
calories 64, fat 3g, saturated fat 2g, cholesterol 8mg, carbohydrates 6g, fiber 1g, protein 2g, sodium 78mg

Paprika Mushroom Appetizer

Preparation time: 10 minutes
Cooking time: 4 hours
Servings: 2

Ingredients:
pound mushroom caps
1 yellow onion, chopped
3 garlic cloves, minced
1 cup veggie stock
tablespoon heavy cream
teaspoons smoked paprika
Salt and black pepper to the taste
tablespoons parsley, chopped

Directions:
In your slow cooker, mix mushrooms with garlic, onion, stock and paprika, stir, cover and cook on High for 4 hours.
Add parsley, coconut cream, salt and pepper, toss, arrange on a platter and serve them as an appetizer.
Enjoy!

Nutrition:
Calories 300, Fat 6g, Fiber 12g, Carbs 16g, Protein 6g

Romano and Asiago Cheese Crisps

Preparation time: 15 minutes
Cooking time: 30 minutes
Servings: 8

Ingredients:
1¼ cups Romano cheese, grated
½ cup Asiago cheese, grated
2 ripe tomatoes, peeled
½ teaspoon sea salt
½ teaspoon chili powder
1 teaspoon dried oregano
1 teaspoon dried basil
1 teaspoon dried parsley flakes
1 teaspoon garlic powder

Directions:
Mix the cheese in a bowl. Place tablespoon-sized heaps of the mixture onto parchmentlined baking pans.

Bake in the preheated oven at 380°F (193°C) approximately 7 minutes until beginning to brown around the edges.

Let them stand for about 15 minutes until crisp.

Meanwhile, purée the tomatoes in your food processor. Bring the puréed tomatoes to a simmer, add the remaining ingredients and cook for 30 minutes or until it has thickened and cooked through.

Serve the cheese crisps with the spicy tomato sauce on the side. Bon appétit!

Nutrition:
calories 110, fat 7.5g, protein 8.4g, carbs 2.0g, net carbs 1.6g, fiber 0.4g

Cheese and Ham Egg Cakes

Preparation time: 15 minutes
Cooking time: 25 minutes
Servings: 8

Ingredients:

2 cups ham, chopped

⅓ cup Parmesan cheese, grated

1 tablespoon parsley, chopped

¼ cup almond flour

9 eggs

⅓ cup mayonnaise, sugar-free

¼ teaspoon garlic powder

¼ cup onion, chopped

Sea salt to taste

Cooking spray

Directions:

Preheat your oven to 375°F (190°C). Lightly grease nine muffin pans with cooking spray, and set aside.

Place the onion, ham, garlic powder, and salt, in a food processor, and pulse until ground.

Stir in the mayonnaise, almond flour, and Parmesan cheese. Press this mixture into the muffin cups.

Bake for 5 minutes. Crack an egg into each muffin cup. Return to the oven and bake for 20 more minutes or until the tops are firm to the touch and eggs are cooked. Leave to cool slightly before serving.

Nutrition:

calories 266, fat 18.0g, protein 13.5g, carbs 1.6g, net carbs 1.0g, fiber 0.6g

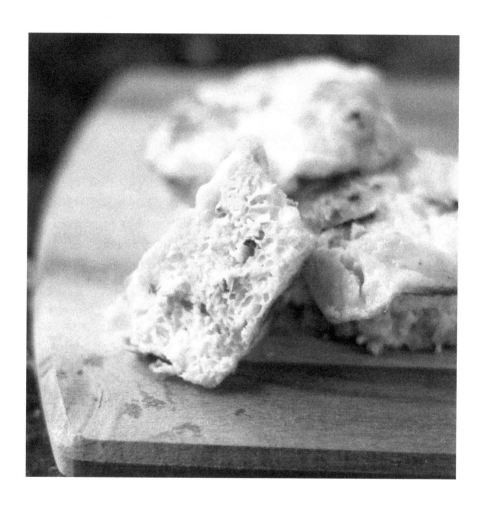

Cream Cheese Mushroom Salsa

Preparation time: 10 minutes
Cooking time: 4 hours
Servings: 2

Ingredients:
cup green bell peppers, chopped
1 small yellow onion, chopped
1 garlic clove, minced
½ pound mushrooms, chopped
12 ounces tomato sauce
¼ cup cream cheese, cubed
Salt and black pepper to the taste

Directions:
In your slow cooker, mix bell peppers with onion, garlic, mushrooms, tomato sauce, cheese, salt and pepper, stir, cover and cook on Low for 4 hours. Divide into bowls and serve as a party salsa with crackers on the side. Enjoy!

Nutrition:
calories 285, fat 4g, fiber 7g, carbs 12g, protein 4g

Dessert

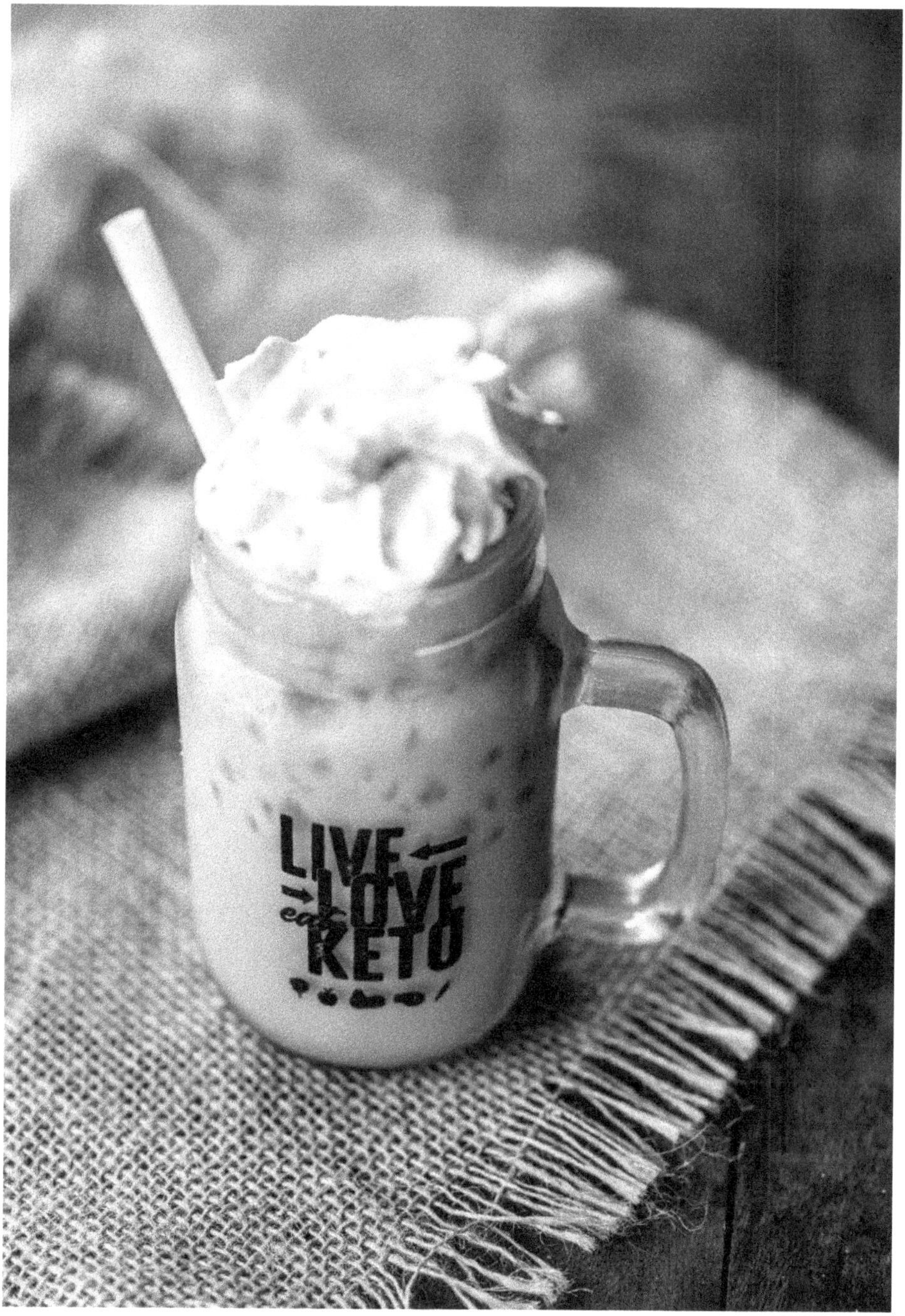
LIVE
LOVE
eat
KETO

Sesame Cookies

Preparation Time: 15 minutes
Cooking Time: 15 minutes
Servings: 12

Ingredients:
1/3 cup monk fruit sweetener, granulated
3/4 teaspoon baking powder
1 cup almond flour
1 egg
1 teaspoon toasted sesame oil
1/2 cup grass-fed butter, at room temperature
1/2 cup sesame seeds

Directions:
Let the oven heat up to 350F.
The dry ingredients must be combined in a bowl. The wet ingredients must be mixed in a separate bowl. Pour the wet mixture into the bowl for the dry ingredients. Stir until the mixture has a thick consistency and forms a dough. Put the sesame seeds in a third bowl. Divide and shape the dough into 16 11/2-inch balls, then dunk the balls in the bowl of sesame seeds to coat well. Bash the balls until they are 1/2 inch thick, then put them on a baking sheet lined with parchment paper.
Keep a little space between each of them. Baking Time (15 minutes). Remove the cookies from the oven and allow to cool for a few minutes before serving.

Nutrition:
calories 174, fat 12.4g, fiber 12.5g, carbohydrates 8.5 g, protein 6.8g

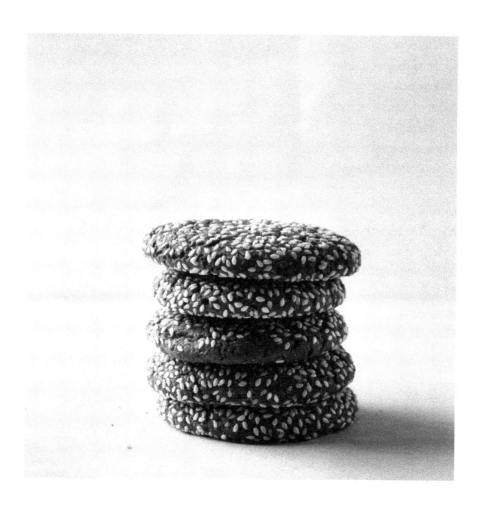

Creamy Rhubarb and Plums Bowls

Preparation time: 10 minutes
Cooking time: 2 hours
Servings: 2

Ingredients:
1 cup plums, pitted and halved
1 cup rhubarb, sliced
1 cup coconut cream
½ teaspoon vanilla extract
½ cup sugar
½ tablespoon lemon juice
1 teaspoon almond extract

Directions:
In your slow cooker, mix the plums with the rhubarb, cream and the other ingredients, toss, put the lid on and cook on High for 2 hours.
Divide the mix into bowls and serve.

Nutrition:
calories 162, fat 2g, fiber 2g, carbs 4g, protein 5g

Candied Lemon

Preparation time: 20 minutes
Cooking time: 4 hours
Servings: 4

Ingredients:
5 lemons, peeled and cut into medium segments
3 cups white sugar
3 cups water

Directions:
In your slow cooker, mix lemons with sugar and water, cover, cook on Low for 4 hours, transfer them to bowls and serve cold.

Nutrition:
calories 62, fat 3g, fiber 5g, carbs 3g, protein 4g

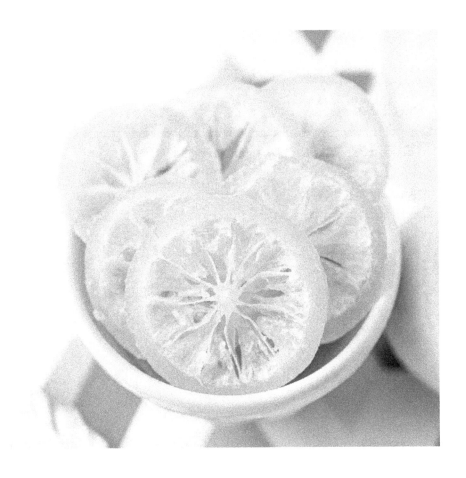

Pear Crumble

Preparation time: 10 minutes
Cooking time: 3 hours
Servings: 2

Ingredients:
4 tablespoons oatmeal
pear, chopped
tablespoons sugar
1 tablespoon coconut oil
½ teaspoon ground cardamom
1 tablespoon dried apricots, chopped
¼ cup of coconut milk

Directions:
Mix oatmeal with chopped pear, sugar, coconut oil, ground cardamom, dried apricots, and coconut milk.
Then put the mixture in the slow cooker and close the lid.
Cook the crumble on Low for 3 hours.

Nutrition:
255 calories, 2.4g protein, 32g carbohydrates, 14.8g fat, 4.1g fiber, 0mg cholesterol, 6mg sodium, 215mg potassium

Coconut Brownies

Preparation time: 10 minutes
Cooking time: 20 minutes
Servings: 10

Ingredients:
½ cup butter, melted
1¼ cups coconut flour
1 teaspoon baking powder
⅓ cup cocoa powder, unsweetened
1 cup Xylitol

Directions:
Mix all ingredients in the order listed above.

Scrape the batter into a parchment-lined baking pan.

Bake in the preheated oven at 360°F (182°C) approximately 20 minutes or until a tester comes out clean.

Transfer to a cooling rack for 1 hour before slicing and serving. Bon appétit!

Nutrition:
Calories 124, fat 12.8g, protein 0.8g, carbs 3.2g, net carbs 1.4g, fiber 1.8g

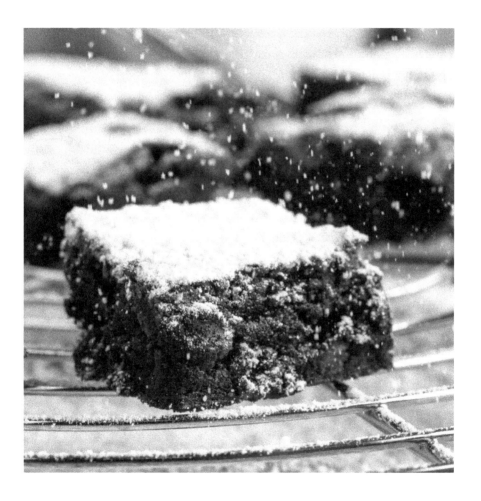

Cinnamon Cream Cheese Mousse

Preparation time: 15 minutes
Cooking time: 0 minutes
Servings: 8

Ingredients:

2 ounces (57 g) full-fat cream cheese, at room temperature

1½ cups heavy whipping cream, divided

¼ cup granulated erythritol–monk fruit blend;

less sweet: 2 tablespoons

½ teaspoon vanilla extract

½ teaspoon salt

½ cup finely milled almond flour

¼ cup coconut flour

¼ cup granulated erythritol–monk fruit blend

½ teaspoon ground cinnamon

⅛ teaspoon sea salt

4 tablespoons (½ stick) cold unsalted butter, thinly sliced

Directions:

Put the large metal bowl in the freezer to chill for at least 5 minutes. In the large chilled bowl, using an electric mixer on medium high, mix the cream cheese and ¼ cup of heavy cream until well combined. Add the erythritol–monk fruit blend, vanilla, and salt and mix until just combined. Add the remaining 1¼ cups of heavy cream and beat on high for about 3 minutes, until stiff peaks form, stopping and scraping the bowl once or twice, as needed. Refrigerate for at least 1 hour and up to overnight before serving.

In the small bowl, combine the almond flour, coconut flour, erythritol–monk fruit blend, cinnamon, and salt. Add the sliced butter and combine using a fork until the mixture resembles coarse crumbs. Set aside until ready to serve. Serve the mousse in short glasses or small mason jars topped with the crumble. Store leftovers in an airtight container for up to 5 days in the refrigerator.

Nutrition: (½ Cup)
calories 274, fat 28.9g, protein 3.1g, carbs 3.1g, net carbs 1.9g, fiber 1.2g

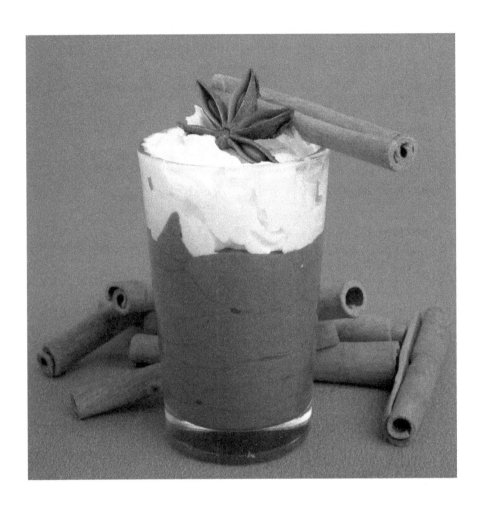

Lavender Cookies

Preparation time: 20 minutes
Cooking time: 2 hours
Servings: 6

Ingredients:
1 teaspoon lavender extract
1 teaspoon vanilla extract
1 cup coconut flour
¼ cup butter
1 egg, whisked
1 teaspoon baking powder
½ teaspoon olive oil

Directions:
Mix the lavender extract and vanilla extract.
Add the coconut flour and butter.
Add the whisked egg and baking powder.
Knead into a smooth dough.
Roll out the dough and cut the cookies with a cookie cutter.
Pour the olive oil in the slow cooker.
Transfer the cookies to the slow cooker and cook them for 2 hours on High.
Cool the cookies and serve!

Nutrition:
calories 165, fat 10.8g, fiber 8g, carbs 13.9g, protein 3.7g

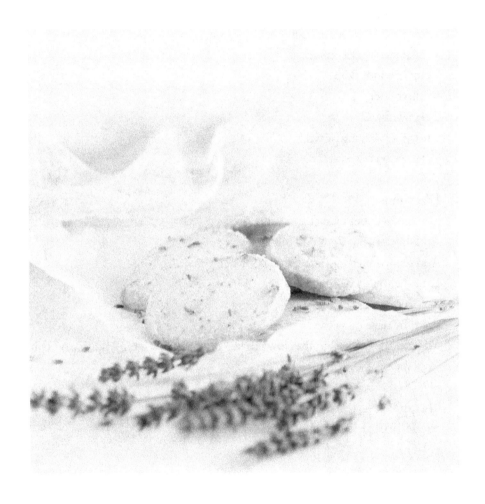

Other Keto Recipes

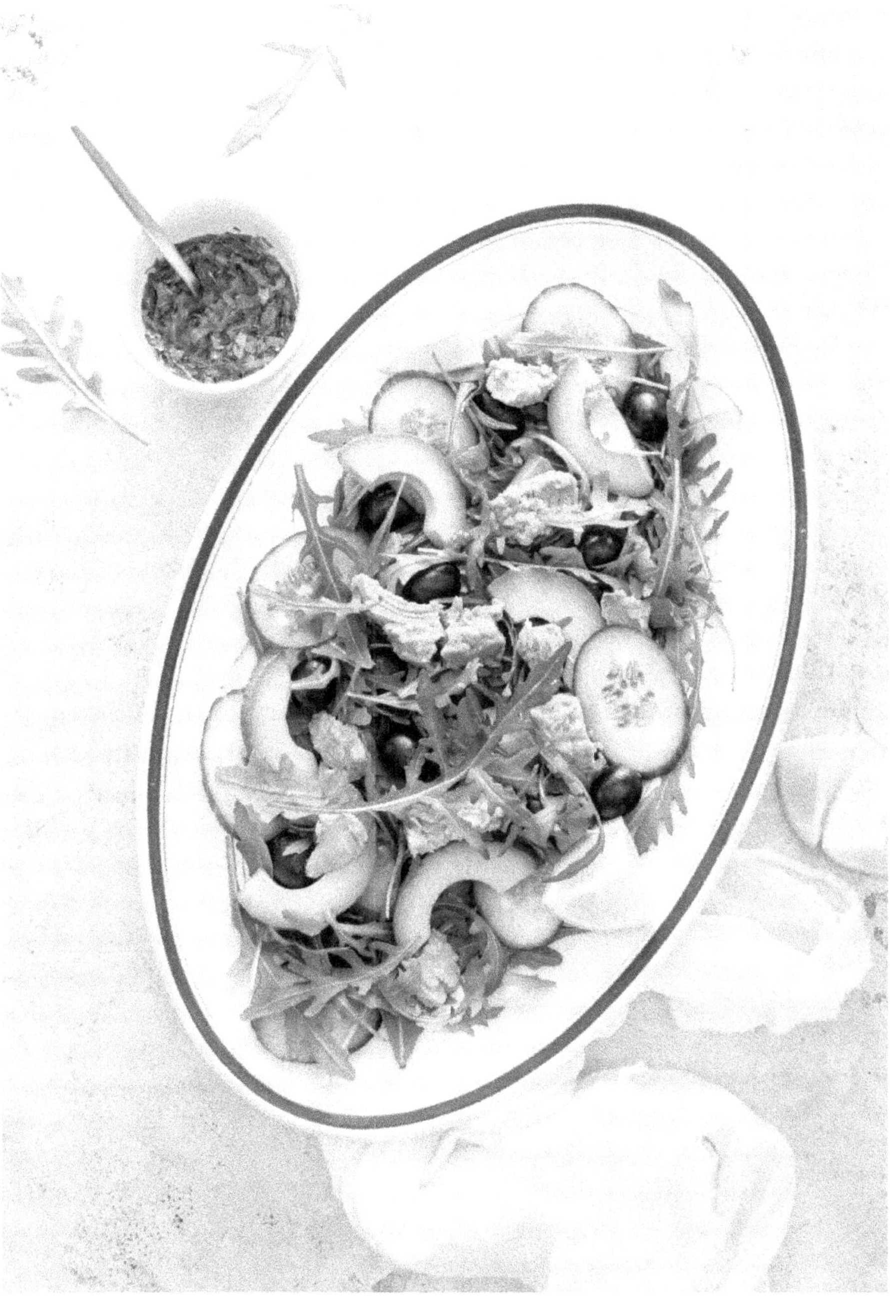

Bread with Bananas and Almonds

Preparation time: 10 minutes
Cooking time: 4 hours
Servings: 2

Ingredients:
egg
tablespoons butter, melted
½ cup sugar
cup flour
½ teaspoon baking powder
¼ teaspoon baking soda
A pinch of cinnamon powder
A pinch of nutmeg, ground
bananas, mashed
¼ cup almonds, sliced
Cooking Spray

Directions:
In a bowl, mix sugar with flour, baking powder, baking soda, cinnamon and nutmeg and stir. Add egg, butter, almonds and bananas and stir really well. Grease your slow cooker with cooking spray, pour bread mix, cover and cook on Low for 4 hours.
Slice bread and serve for breakfast. Enjoy!

Nutrition:
calories 211, fat 3g, fiber 6g, carbs 12g, protein 5g

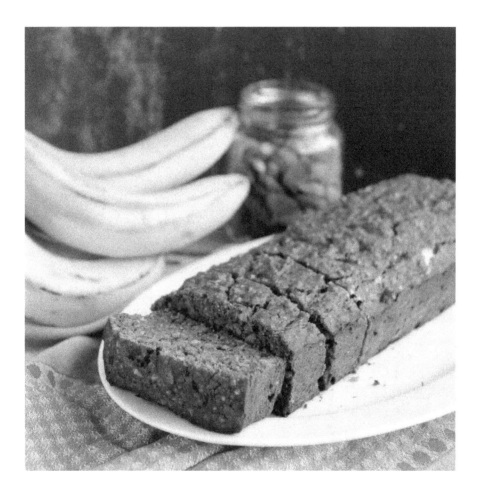

Chicken and Pepper Skewers

Preparation time: 10 minutes
Cooking time: 10 minutes
Servings: 6

Ingredients:
2 tablespoons olive oil
4 tablespoons dry sherry
tablespoon stone-ground mustard
1½ pounds (680 g) chicken, skinless, boneless and cubed
red onions, cut into wedges
1 green bell pepper, cut into 1-inch pieces
1 red bell pepper, cut into 1-inch pieces
1 yellow bell pepper, cut into 1-inch pieces
½ teaspoon sea salt
¼ teaspoon ground black pepper, or more to taste

Directions:
In a mixing bowl, combine the olive oil, dry sherry, mustard and chicken until well coated.
Alternate skewering the chicken and vegetables until you run out of ingredients. Season with salt and black pepper.
Preheat your grill to medium-high heat.
Place the kabobs on the grill, flipping every 2 minutes and cook to desired doneness. Serve warm.

Nutrition:
calories: 201, fat: 8.2g, protein: 24.3g, carbs:7.0g, net carbs: 5.7g, fiber: 1.3g

Beef and Cheese Rolls

Preparation Time: 10 minutes
Cooking Time: 20 minutes
Servings: 4

Ingredients:
 2 tbsp. vegetable oil, divided
large onion, thinly sliced
large bell peppers, thinly sliced
1 tsp. dried oregano
Kosher salt
Freshly ground black pepper
1 lb. skirt steak, thinly sliced
1 c. shredded provolone
8 large butterhead lettuce leaves
2tbsp. freshly chopped parsley

Directions:

Heat 1 tbsp. oil and put chopped onion and sliced bell peppers and sprinkle with oregano, salt, and pepper. Cook, often stirring, until the onion and pepper are tender, about 3-5 minutes. Transfer the cooked peppers and onions to a plate and add the remaining oil in the skillet. Put the steak in the skillet and spread a single layer, season with salt and pepper.

Sear until the steak is seared on one side, about 2-3 minutes. Flip and sear on the second side until cooked through, about 2-3 minutes more for medium. Put the cooked and pepper back to skillet and mix to combine. Sprinkle the cheese over onions and steak. Cover the steak skillet with a lid and cook until the cheese has melted, turn off the heat. Lay the lettuce leaves on a serving platter. Top with steak mixture on each piece of lettuce. Garnish with parsley and serve warm.

Nutrition:

calories 375, fat 15.1g, fiber 12.9g, carbohydrates 4.3 g, protein 17.5g

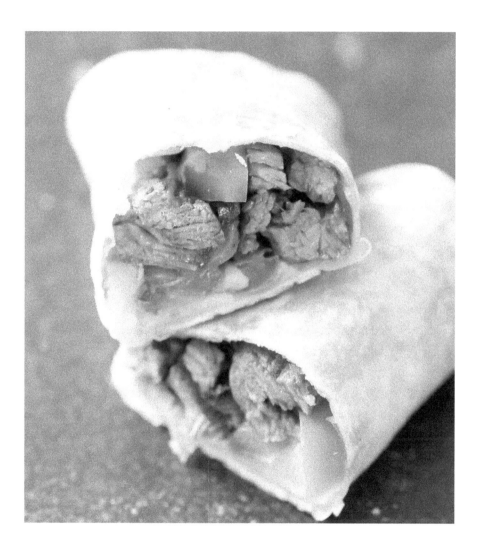

Beef Gratin

Preparation time: 15 minutes
Cooking time: 40 minutes
Servings: 5

Ingredients:

2 teaspoons onion flakes
2 pounds (907 g) ground beef
2 garlic cloves, minced
Salt and black pepper, to taste
cup Mozzarella cheese, shredded
cups Fontina cheese, shredded
cup Russian dressing
tablespoons sesame seeds, toasted
20 dill pickle slices
1 iceberg lettuce head, torn

Directions:

Set a pan over medium heat, place in beef, garlic, salt, onion flakes, and pepper, and cook for 5 minutes. Remove to a baking dish, stir in Russian dressing, Mozzarella, and spread 1 cup of the Fontina cheese.

Lay the pickle slices on top, spread over the remaining Fontina cheese and sesame seeds, place in the oven at 350°F (180°C), and bake for 20 minutes. Arrange the lettuce on a serving platter and top with the gratin.

Nutrition:

calories 585, fat 48.1g, protein 40.9g, carbs 8.5g, net carbs 5.2g, fiber 3.3g

Tacos with Tilapia and Cabbage

Preparation time: 10 minutes
Cooking time: 5 minutes
Servings: 4

Ingredients:
1 tablespoon olive oil
teaspoon chili powder
tilapia fillets
1 teaspoon paprika
4 keto tortillas
Slaw:
½ cup red cabbage, shredded
1 tablespoon lemon juice
1 teaspoon apple cider vinegar
1 tablespoon olive oil

Directions:
Season tilapia with chili powder and paprika. Heat the olive oil in a skillet over medium heat. Add tilapia, and cook until blackened, about 3 minutes per side. Cut into strips. Divide the tilapia between the tortillas. Combine all of the slaw ingredients in a bowl. Divide the slaw between the tortillas.

Nutrition:
calories 261, fat 20.1g, protein 13.9g, carbs 5.5g, net carbs 3.6g, fiber 1.9g

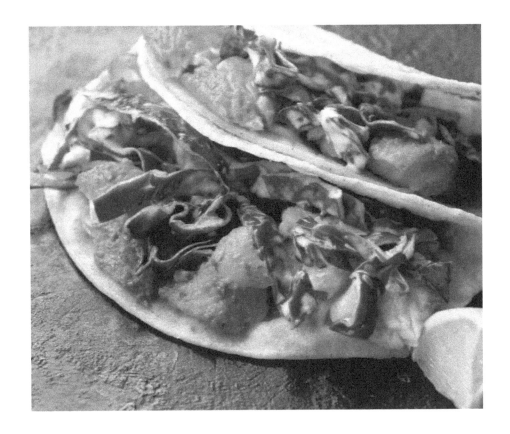

Salad with Capers in Greek Style

Preparation time: 10 minutes
Cooking time: 0 minutes
Servings: 4

Ingredients:

5 tomatoes, chopped
1 large cucumber, chopped
1 green bell pepper, chopped
1 small red onion, chopped
16 Kalamata olives, chopped
4 tablespoons capers
7 ounces (198 g) Feta cheese, chopped
1 teaspoon oregano, dried
4 tablespoons olive oil
Salt to taste

Directions:

Place tomatoes, pepper, cucumber, onion, Feta and olives in a bowl. Mix to combine. Season with salt. Combine the capers, olive oil and oregano in a small bowl. Drizzle the dressing over the salad.

Nutrition:

calories 324, fat 27.8g, protein 9.4g, carbs 11.9g, net carbs 8.0g, fiber 3.9g

Soup with Beef and Herbs

Prepation time: 15 minutes
Cooking time: 40 minutes
Servings: 6

Ingredients:
1 pound (454 g) beef chuck roast, cubed
6 cups beef bone broth (you can also use regular beef broth)
yellow onion, chopped
cloves garlic, chopped
2 carrots, chopped
2 stalks celery, sliced
1 teaspoon fresh thyme, chopped
½ teaspoon dried oregano
1 handful fresh basil, chopped
Salt and pepper, to taste
1 tablespoon coconut oil, for cooking

Directions:
Add the coconut oil to a skillet and brown the beef over medium heat.
Add the beef and the remaining ingredients minus the basil to a stockpot and bring to a boil.
Reduce to a simmer and cook for about 30 minutes or until the vegetables are tender.
Serve with freshly chopped basil.

Nutrition:
calories 220, fat 9.0g, protein 29.0g, carbs 6.0g, net carbs 5.0g, fiber 1.0g

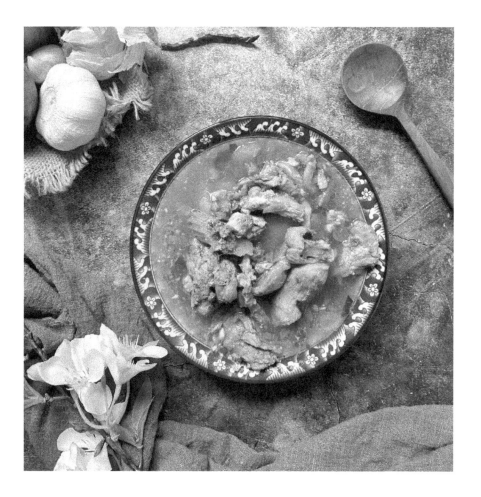

Zucchini and Bacon Meatballs

Preparation Time: 3 hrs.
Cooking Time: 20 minutes
Servings: 10

Ingredients:
2 zucchinis, shredded
2 bacon slices, chopped
1/2 cup cream cheese, at room temperature
1 cup fontina cheese
1/4 cup capers
1 clove garlic, crushed
1/2 cup grated Parmesan cheese
1/2 tsp. poppy seeds
1/4 tsp. dried dill weed
1/2 tsp. onion powder
Salt and black pepper, to taste
1 cup crushed pork rinds

Directions:
Preheat oven to 360 F.
Thoroughly mix zucchinis, capers, 1/2 of Parmesan cheese, garlic, cream cheese, bacon, and fontina cheese until well combined. Shape the mixture into balls. Refrigerate for 3 hours. In a mixing bowl, mix the remaining Parmesan cheese, crushed pork rinds, dill, black pepper, onion powder, poppy seeds, and salt. Roll cheese ball in Parmesan mixture to coat. Arrange in a greased baking dish in a single layer and bake in the oven for 15-20 minutes, shaking once.

Nutrition:
calories 227, fat 12.5g, fiber 9.4g carbohydrates 4.3 g

Crunchy Kale

Preparation time: 15 minutes
Cooking time: 15 minutes
Servings; 2

Ingredients:

2 cups kale, torn into pieces

1 tablespoons olive oil

Sea salt, to taste

¼ teaspoon pepper

½ teaspoon onion powder ½ teaspoon garlic powder

½ teaspoon fresh dill, minced

½ tablespoon fresh parsley, minced

Start by preheating your oven to 320°F (160°C).

Directions:

Toss the kale leaves with all other ingredients until well coated. Bake for 10 to 14 minutes, depending on how crisp you like them.

Store the kale chips in an airtight container for up to a week. Bon appétit!

Nutrition:

calories 69, fat 6.5g, protein 0.5g, carbs 1.5g, net carbs 1.0g, fiber 0.5g

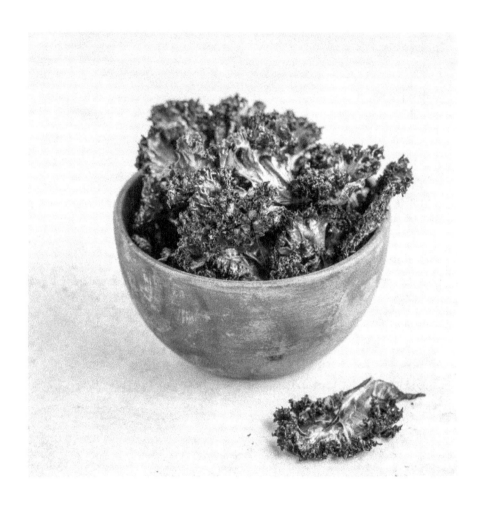

Apple Pie

Preparation Time: 15 minutes
Cooking Time: 25 minutes
Servings: 6

Ingredients:

6 tbsp. butter

2 cups almond flour

½ tsp. cinnamon

1/3 cup sweetener Filling:

2 cups sliced Granny Smith

1/4 cup butter

1/4 cup sweetener

1/2 tsp. cinnamon

1/2 tsp. lemon juice

Topping:

1/4 tsp. cinnamon

2 tbsp. sweetener

Directions:

Preheat oven to 370°F and combine all crust ingredients in a bowl. Press this mixture into the bottom of a greased pan. Bake for 5 minutes.

Meanwhile, combine the apples and lemon juice in a bowl and sit until the crust is ready.

Arrange them on top of the crust.

Combine remaining filling ingredients, and brush this mixture over the apples. Bake for about 30 minutes.

Press the apples down with a spatula, return to oven, and bake for 20 more minutes. Combine the cinnamon and sweetener in a bowl, and sprinkle over the tart.

Nutrition:

calories 276, fat 11g, fiber 10.4g, carbohydrates 2.1g, Protein: 3.1g

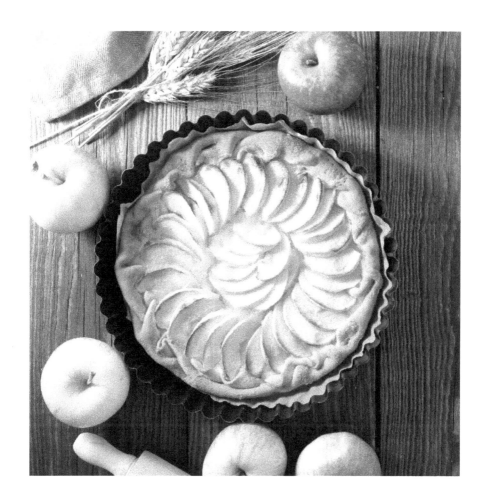